Praise for *Brainhacker*

"Memory expert David Farrow gives readers memory-smartening tools that can last a lifetime. Its reader-friendly format, personal stories, and engaging humor is just what the brain's memory centers like. *Brainhacker* is a memory book for all ages, from high-school and college students when memories are maturing to seniors when memories are fading. Read it, do it, and remember it!"

—William Sears, MD, author of *The Healthy Brain Book*

"Interwoven with Dave Farrow's personal narrative, *Brainhacker* is a spritely, informative blitz through brain science. His hacks are handy, helpful tools for improving yourself and your lifestyle."

—Marc Milstein, PhD, author of *The Age-Proof Brain*

BRAINHACKER

BRAINHACKER

BRAINHACKER

Master **MEMORY, FOCUS, EMOTIONS**, and More to Unleash the Genius Within

DAVE FARROW

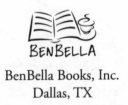

BenBella Books, Inc.
Dallas, TX

BenBella Books, Inc.
10440 N. Central Expressway
Suite 800
Dallas, TX 75231
benbellabooks.com
Send feedback to feedback@benbellabooks.com

BenBella is a federally registered trademark.

Printed in the United States of America
10 9 8 7 6 5 4 3 2 1

Library of Congress Control Number: 2022945989
ISBN 9781637741405 (print)
ISBN 9781637741412 (ebook)

Illustrations by Ralph Voltz
Text design and composition by PerfecType, Nashville, TN
Cover design by Sarah Avinger
Cover image © Shutterstock / Zaie (brain lineart); Adobe Stock / Soho A studio
Printed by Lake Book Manufacturing

This book is dedicated to my parents, sister, friends Jo and Scott, and a great teacher, Mr. Muller. Rest in peace, sir. You saw the potential in me, and that made all the difference in the world. I hope this book helps to fulfill your dying wish: to give the gift of memory to others. You won't be forgotten.

THIS IS REAL.

The strategies you're about to read have been tested by thousands of students. The events are real, although some events have been dramatized, combined, or edited for improved readability. Some names have been changed for privacy . . . but these people know who they are.

CONTENTS

INTRODUCTION: HOW TO USE THIS BOOK

You probably picked up this book because you heard about my journey from ADHD and dyslexic kid with chronic pain to Guinness record holder for memory and beyond. When I struggled with these challenges, everyone told me, "There is no manual to run the brain."

Not anymore.

The goal of *Brainhacker* is to be the manual for your brain. Or at least, the first volume in the journey. In this book I intend to show you how to unlock the superhuman abilities we all possess.

Examples include:

- Memorizing any amount of information
- Triggering perfect focus at will
- Learning eight times faster than anyone else
- Speed-reading
- Stopping self-sabotage
- Ending food cravings
- Truly fighting age-related mental decline
- Editing your own habits
- Lip-reading

We start simple, and then stack skills Voltron-like to form amazing, complex powers. Each hack is then summarized at the end of the chapter.

But I want this to be more than a list of tricks. I've included many stories of my life here, and I want you to follow along with my process of learning or creating hacks, and then apply my hacks to your life. But I want you to be empowered to make your own brain hacks too. That's right: I am not the guru with all the answers. I think I can help you solve a great many things with what I know, but what is more powerful is learning the process of making hacks yourself.

In fact, let's start right now with our first brainhack. Stories help us remember and understand difficult concepts and new information, which is another reason why I have included many moments of my life here. Stories help us to experience the concepts rather than just get a summary of the bullet points.

The Story Hack

Stories help make the lessons stick and show you how to make new brainhacks yourself. If you skip the story and jump right to the summaries of the hacks, you miss out on how the brainhack was created and that context helps us learn.

Humans are storytelling creatures for a reason. Learning through stories works because your brain is given context and can imagine the events in a personal, highly memorable manner.

And that is your first brainhack. Your journey has begun.

THE BODY-MIND CONNECTION

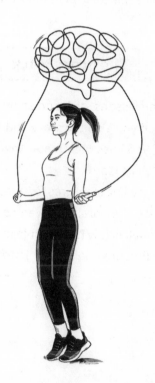

Nearly every action in the body influences the brain. When our mind is stuck in patterns, blanking out, overtired, hyperactive, or emotional, it can be impossible to think your way out of anything. Instead, hack your brain by moving your body.

1 | The Body-Brainhack

I can never spell *dyslexia* without looking it up.

I have a theory that when they named this condition, they made it hard to spell on purpose as a cruel joke on us. Think about it, how many words have an X in the middle?

When they labeled me ADD/ADHD, they knew what they were doing, though. It's only a few letters—perfect if you don't have any attention span to speak of.

As I sat in the dining room in my pajamas, trying my best to motivate my six-and-a-half-year-old son to read, I couldn't help but feel silly. I was known for being a Guinness record-holder for memory, a CEO, a brain expert, and a bestselling author—the person who turned ADHD and dyslexia into advantages—and yet, at that moment, I would be thrilled if I could get my son to pay attention for five seconds. Being a dad is my favorite role, but on this day, it felt like a chore.

We were sitting at the table and looking down at phonics flashcards. And for the last ten minutes, we'd been working on sounding out the words. Yet, it wasn't going well. Lex couldn't stop goofing around—or so I thought.

And when I couldn't take it any longer, I snapped. "Lex! You know how to sound this out, so why are you goofing around so much?" I held the card up to his face.

"I'm trying, but I don't know . . ."

He paused, and we both looked up as my wife entered the room. When I turned back to him, I saw that the clowning face was broken as a single tear slid down his cheek. Moments later, he couldn't hold it back, and the tears flowed. I dropped the card and pulled him into a hug.

"Buddy boo, what is it?" I asked, feeling like a royal ass at that moment.

He continued to cry as he wrapped his legs and arms around me, as any vulnerable six-year-old would. I held on and waited patiently until he caught his breath.

"I'm trying to focus," he sniffed, "but it's hard. I don't know, but if it's a *b* sound or a *d* sound, it changes in my head." In between gasps, he pointed at the flashcard I had thrown down: *bottle*.

My gut tensed with pain. I had to overcome ADHD and dyslexia challenges as a child. Heck, as an adult, I'd lectured on it, coached, and guided thousands of students on how to turn that challenge into an advantage. But this was the first time it'd ever hit so close to home. In that moment, I realized my son was maybe too much of a chip off the old block.

"You mean you reverse the letters in your head?" I asked.

"No, I'm reading *forward*, not like, in *reverse*," he replied, shaking his head at me. "Duh."

With that, the tension broke. His adorable response threw me into a fit of laughter, and Lex followed along, even though he didn't know why. It felt good. After the brief laugh though, his sad face returned. His shoulders were hunched forward, sulking while looking down.

"Let's change gears," I told him.

I stood up and took a deep breath and prompted him to follow along. I mimed a soldier marching with my head held high. We puffed out our chests and held our chins up. I even made a goofy face, and it got a laugh.

"When you feel emotional or sad," I explained, "your body will follow your brain and start to withdraw from the world."

Happy Brains, Please Stand Up!: The Smile Brainhack

Our minds and bodies are connected so closely that our thoughts influence our heart rate, blood pressure, and even immune response. The reverse is also true: By simply smiling or laughing, we can lower blood pressure and better fight disease.

This mind-body connection was once thought of as a pseudoscience, but it is now an established fact. Subjects who are simply told to laugh, smile, or change posture on a daily basis have shown surprising mental and health improvements, from lowering depression, raising test scores, and even strengthening immune responses to disease. This should not be used as a tool to mask or ignore underlying causes of conditions like depression or anxiety; instead, therapists use this phenomenon as a tool to temporarily improve moods in patients so they have more strength to tackle the underlying issues involved—and brainhackers sometimes use it to help their kids finish their homework.

Friendly note to men: Smiling may be good for the brain, but telling a woman you don't know to smile may not go over well.

I explained how his body was slumped forward and his head was down looking at the ground. This posture told his brain to stay sad. But it goes both ways. If we want to feel better, we can shake off these bad feelings by moving our bodies.

After a few minutes of standing and smiling, my son was feeling better but was still fidgeting a bit. Changing how your body moves can instantly shift moods and emotions in the brain. But if we want bigger change, we need to balance brain chemistry.

Take a Walk Brainhack

The brain is the most powerful computer with the worst battery. We can go from a deep flow state of focus and clarity to feeling clumsy and forgetful in minutes.

The brain could be the most complex thing in the known universe, but we can't tap into the power of that tool without understanding how it runs.

You will learn later in this book (page 123) how quickly our brains run out of focus power. This is a feature and not a bug in the system. The brain takes a lot of energy to function, so it is perfectly tuned for short moments of extreme challenge and long periods of leisure, much like we would find if we lived in the wild.

Just thinking about a difficult subject can raise serotonin and glutamate, according to multiple studies, thus triggering sleepiness. That means, oddly, that thinking hard can make it difficult to continue to think hard. But there is a simple hack: Move!

Serotonin binds with oxygen, so any aerobic exercise will clear it out of the brain. Glutamate and the other byproducts of overthinking also balance out when we exercise. This is where we get the age-old phrase, "I took a walk to clear my head."

I challenged Lex to race me around the kitchen amid protests from my better half. It only took three laps to get the result. Clear head and no fidgeting. Not only does a little physical exercise balance the brain, but it's also great for ADHD.

CHAPTER **SUMMARY**

- The Smile Brainhack: Every mental state has a corresponding physical expression. We smile and laugh when happy, stand tall when confident, and look down and hunch our shoulders when sad. By adopting one of these physical shapes, we can affect our mental state. Laughter therapy has become popular because of this.

- Take a Walk Brainhack: When we enter a mental challenge like a study session, our brain chemistry is balanced. Cognitive work throws this out of balance. The good news is that even light aerobic movement like walking rebalances the brain, quickly clearing your head and allowing you to get back to the task refreshed. Many great thinkers take afternoon walks to improve performance.

2 | The Tale of Two Breaths

Back at the table, I ask my son, "Quick quiz, Lex. Can you remember the names of the planets?"

Of course, I already knew that he could; he loved the hard sciences. But he didn't look confident. He wasn't quite over the crying session, and I could see that my question was making him nervous about making another mistake. (Sometimes I forget how much little things feel like the end of the world to kids.)

I changed tack. "Okay, we just did the Smile (page 7) and Take a Walk (page 8) Brainhacks. But to get the best memory recall, let's do one more body brainhack."

"Yes," he beamed, excited to learn my secrets.

* * *

There are two nervous systems in the body: the automatic and autonomic (also called the sympathetic and parasympathetic, or simply the subconscious and conscious). Nearly every part of your body has picked a side of this system. When you think of lifting your hand, it goes up. Think about moving your feet, and they move. But parts like your heart, sweat glands, blood vessels, and even your pupils (when they dilate, for example) are run by the subconscious system. This is great because your heart will keep beating without any effort from you. But one organ is a double agent: your lungs. They will expand and contract exactly to your wishes, but when you don't think about it, your brain takes over and makes sure you keep breathing. Also a good thing.

So by controlling your breathing you can tell your body's subconscious system to act in different ways. This is the reason the lungs are a special tool in the mind-body connection. Slow your breathing and you relax, speed it up and you stress out. With practice, you can essentially turn your stress and relaxation responses off and on. If you want to know why, the reason is as old as nature.

When humans were just nomadic hunters exposed to the wild, they had to develop ways to trigger their stress reaction to danger. Think about what people look like when they are surprised or scared. You probably imagine them opening their mouth and taking in a big gulp of air and even lifting their elbows away from their body to maximize lung capacity. This reaction prepares them for the fight that will come soon. In the same way, if we breathe quick, short breaths, we are essentially telling our body to freak out. The stress response makes your chest move up and down, and you become temporarily dumb from blood rushing away from the brain to the vital organs and muscles in preparation for the fight-or-flight reaction to come. So if you panic on test-taking day, you will score well below your potential, simply because your body thinks this test is actually a tiger about to eat you. Even if there is no direct danger, the body still tries to prepare for a fight.

So, if we can trigger stress, can we also trigger relaxation?

Yes.

I told Lex about the two different body systems, and we did an exercise to feel the difference. We placed one hand on our chest and the other on our stomach. After a few minutes, it was clear he was breathing with his chest and getting more and more stressed.

After closing his eyes to focus, his chest slowed down and stopped as the stomach took over movement. Three breaths later, he opened his eyes and smiled confidently.

Baby Breath Brainhack

Think of how a relaxed baby sleeps. I remember seeing my sleeping child's stomach moving in and out like a balloon while his chest was frozen in place. That's the secret: Chest breathing (when your chest moves up and down) supports the stress response, and belly breathing (when your stomach moves in and out) triggers calm.

Step One: Put one hand on your chest and the other on your stomach.

Step Two: Breathe while noticing which hand moves the most.

Step Three: Breathe so the top hand is motionless, and the stomach hand moves the most. Take deeper and deeper breaths, and make it a habit. Train your body to react to stress with relaxation.

"Okay, starting from the sun," he began excitedly reciting the planets, waving his hands like a conductor greeting his orchestra, "Mercury, Venus, Earth, Mars, the asteroid belt, Jupiter, Saturn, Uranus . . ."

He pronounced Uranus exactly how you'd imagine a six-year-old would.

". . . Aaaaaaaaaaaaaaaaand." He stopped, stumped. "I don't remember." A hint of disappointment crossed his face.

Needing to keep him positive, I pulled out my final and favorite body-brainhack.

"Look up, Lex," I suggested, as I looked up myself.

"When we forget something, we tend to look down because it stresses us out. But our memory works better when we look up.

"So, looking up then sends more energy to the cerebral cortex," I geek-splained to Lex.

While absorbing this information, he looked up at the ceiling while asking himself what came after Uranus. Moments later, a large smile returned to his face.

Look Up Brainhack

Everyone has had an experience where, by instinct, our eyes point to the sky when asked a question. This doesn't mean the memory was written in the clouds. It's just our natural reaction when trying to recall a memory. However, in moments when we're put on the spot, our mind blanks out, and a stress trigger is sent to our brain, which subsequently causes us to look down.

My theory is that recall was difficult for our brains earlier in our evolution, so we started looking up to block out distractions.

"Neptune! And the Kuiper belt."

"And Pluto," added my wife, Dre, with a smile.

"That's not a planet anymore, Mommy!" rebutted Lex, wagging a finger at her.

My wife just shrugged.

"I grew up with Pluto on the list, and it will always be a planet to me," she replied, matter-of-factly.

"Well then, Eris from the Kuiper belt would be a planet too, because it's just about as big," he replied, turning to me with a big grin, "and I didn't even have to look up to know that!"

I laughed.

Lex thought for a moment, thinking of a question. "Daddy, tell me what the eye and the breathing trick is called?"

"It's called a *brainhack*," I explained, looking into his curious eyes. "It's a technique or a way of thinking that gives us a mental ability we didn't have before. Just about anything you could want to do with your brain can be improved with brainhacks."

He jumped into my arms unprompted, saying, "I want to learn all the brainhacks, Daddy."

I paused, enjoying the hug.

"I was just like you, Lex," I continued, hugging him tighter. "I'd do the same thing with the letters, reversing them, and I also had difficulty concentrating without fidgeting, just like you do. But I went on a quest to learn all the brainhacks to turn these problems into extra abilities."

"Daddy is superhuman, Mommy!" he exclaimed, quoting the TV competition that I'd won.

I remembered the pride on his face when he saw me win the grand prize of $50,000 by memorizing binary code in seconds on the Fox show *Superhuman*.

"You can use brainhacks to get amazing powers," I said, knowing that his favorite topic was superheroes.

This did the trick, and Lex pulled back, looking deep into my eyes.

"Like superpowers?"

"In a way. For example, you might have the same brain wiring as me," I told him. "It can make it difficult to learn at first, but I'll teach you the brainhacks that I know, which can turn those disadvantages into superpowers."

Lex grinned with excitement.

"How did you learn these brainhacks? Teach me!"

I had his attention. Now, it was time to tell him my story.

It was the story of how I turned my biggest challenge into an advantage, and in time, helped thousands of others in the same position. I was fourteen years old, and it all started with one small piece of paper. That piece of paper changed my life.

CHAPTER **SUMMARY**

- With the Baby Breath Brainhack, we breathe with our stomachs, like babies, and that triggers relaxation. When we breathe with our chest moving, our brain stresses out more.
- No one knows *why* it happens—just that the Look Up Brainhack seems to direct more energy to the memory centers of the brain and improves recall according to fMRI (functional MRI) studies.

AXIOM TWO

VISUALIZATION

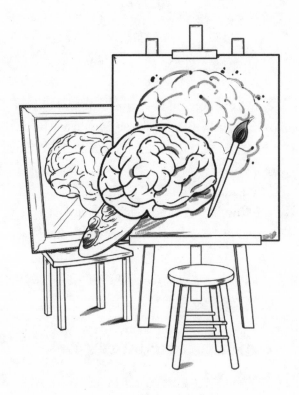

The brain is sitting in the dark painting pictures in our imagination using the paint of our senses. All the data from our senses is organized and contributes to this image we think is real. This mechanism also goes in the other direction. By properly visualizing things in our mind's eye, we can influence the brain to react as if something is really happening.

3 | Where Did I Put My Keys?

"On some level, we can't tell the difference between what is real and imagined."

—Attributed to Socrates as told by Harry Lorayne

The teacher was reading my assessment results on a little slip of paper as the class rolled in. It was the result of one confusing day of testing with a professional to determine if I had learning disabilities. They didn't let me read it yet, but I knew based on what people said that I was ADHD and dyslexic, with hearing problems to boot. After reading this paper, each teacher treated me differently—and not always for the better. Instead of helping me overcome my challenges, it felt like this knowledge lowered the amount of their time I was worth. I felt like a lost cause and needed to get motivated.

But motivation doesn't always come from inspiration or a supportive mentor. I wish that was my story, but my motivation came in the form of a bastard.

My most hated high school class was easy. Too easy.

"All right, everybody listen," Mr. Ross said to the class. "I want to help bring your grades up, but you have to hand something in so I can justify giving you a mark. So, just color in these maps, people."

We were just a month into geography class when it became a coloring and crafts exercise.

"This isn't learning," Becky, a normally quiet girl, said. "I can't believe we're doing this."

"Shut up," scolded Mark, the boy sitting beside her. "Do you want him to give us something hard? Just fill it in, and we get As!"

Becky protested louder this time. "So, this class just started, and you already think we're all failures?"

Others murmured in agreement.

"What's the matter with all of you?" Mr. Ross said, now addressing all the dissenters. "You're in the general level. I'm just trying to make sure you graduate someday."

I could barely keep my eyes open because of the mind-numbing boredom of the class. Later, I discovered that those with ADHD need challenges. The worst thing you can do for an ADHD mind is make things easy. We lose all motivation. Our biggest struggle is internal, getting our brain to care, and we don't care when the stakes are low. Right as I nearly drifted to sleep for the second time, I slipped my hands into my pockets and realized the key to my bike lock was missing.

For the past two weeks, I had lost my key nearly every day. I would leave it in a different place each time. (Another common ADHD trait.) I tried putting it on a necklace or a bracelet, but the string broke. So instead, I tried something else.

* * *

Humans are storytelling creatures because we are visualizing creatures. When someone tells a story, real or fictional, our brain plays it out, at least in part, in our imagination. This is a survival mechanism that allows us to pass on complex information and experiences to others without the same risk.

Because we don't just imagine it either, we experience it. We suspend disbelief and play out the story as if it's happening to us. This is why we can cry, laugh, or even get scared during a movie. We know it's all made up, but our brain thinks it's real. The same mechanism allows us to hack the brain by visualizing anything we want the brain to believe is real. And we can improve our memory by visualizing the unforgettable.

Exploding Keys Brainhack

The key to remembering where you left something is to imagine a very memorable image the second you set down an object. My favorite was to imagine my keys exploding. After a while, I got into the habit of doing this, and it became second nature.

I would set down my stuff and imagine a grenade under it had just made it all go flying across the room. This image would stick even after a long day. The minute I think of these items, the crazy explosion is the first thing that comes to mind, and I recall where I put them.

After realizing my key was missing, I escaped the boredom of the class by diving into my imagination exercise. I thought about my key exploding and took a couple deep breaths. I realized I had set it down in the bathroom for some reason. The location was as clear as day to me, and this time, the exploding image jumped into my mind so fast it shocked me, and I let out a noise.

"What's the matter with you, David? Are you stupid?" Mr. Ross said right to my face.

His blunt question woke me from my trance, and I fixated like a deer in headlights. The entire class stopped and looked at me, and I felt the room spin a bit from embarrassment.

"I'm giving you an easy A. Just take it," he said.

Finally, I spoke up. "I can't focus or even keep my eyes open with this stuff," I answered. "I want to learn things that will help me achieve my goals."

"And what are your goals?" Ross asked with a chuckle.

"I want to run a business, speak on stages, and maybe get into technology and marketing."

I was obsessed with marketing from late night infomercials. My friend Scott's dad had a large collection of infomercial programs, from Tony Robbins to Dale Carnegie. I loved going through them. This was where I first learned memory techniques, and this love made me obsessed with how the programs were marketed.

Still open to possibilities, I asked him, "Can we do something useful like learn flags or the names of countries and capitals?"

To my surprise, several others nodded in approval of this tougher curriculum.

"I read your file, David"—referring to my recent diagnosis—"and I know you can't focus. Your ADHD and dyslexia mean you're not going to run a business. You're probably a kinesthetic learner too. You're not going to work in marketing or technology. I'm just trying to help you graduate. You need to lower your expectations."

My throat tightened up. No words could escape.

"And Becky, what's wrong with you? I mean it. Are you all stupid?" he said, looking around. "You're already in the general level. That's why I'm making it easy for you. I'm the good guy here. If you aim too high in life, you'll just be disappointed. Just color this in, and I can give you extra credit to help you pass this year."

I looked around, judging that about half of the students were smiling like they were getting away with murder. Maybe they struggled in other classes and finally had a way to boost their grades. But the other half were sunk deep into their desks, not laughing or smiling.

When a teacher treats you like you're unteachable, they send a message. You're not worth it. The biggest mistake I made was believing it.

CHAPTER **SUMMARY**

- Visualization Principle: On some level, your brain can't tell the difference between what is real and imagined. This is why you can cry at a movie even though you know that broke character on the screen is actually an actor making millions for their role.

- To memorize an item's location, try the Exploding Keys Brainhack: Imagine something crazy happening to it as you set it down. It can grow tall, come to life, be frozen in a block of ice, or—my favorite— explode. I tested this at McGill University (in association with the National Research Council of Canada) in a double-blind neuro- science study. It showed near-perfect recall among the group that used the technique properly. So, if you love it, blow it up.

4 | Memorable Journeys

After school that day, I went home and cried. I'm not ashamed to admit it. I bawled. Alone in my room for what felt like hours.

I had been pigeonholed by the system—categorized into a stream that didn't fit me. I was told my brain was wrong—that I was broken, stupid, useless. That every instinct and desire I showed to improve myself was either misguided or dangerous.

Wanting a distraction, I headed downstairs to my dad's workshop. He was hunched over an open VCR with an ohmmeter in one hand and the smell of ozone in the air. Our basement looked like a Steve Wozniak garage sale, filled with stacks of TVs, VCRs, and the exciting new devices known as personal computers. But this wasn't a hobby; it was a side business that helped make ends meet. Even with no formal education in this area, he had mastered the ability to fix electronics, literally turning trash into cash.

He would pick up broken TVs and appliances left out on the curb and fix them. The real genius was how he could work his magic on machines from completely different manufacturers.

In those days, when something was broken, people would say it "blew out" because the device often gave off a burning smell that came from a burnt-out resistor or capacitor. The way appliances were built back then, a resistor would literally get so hot it would catch fire for a second, breaking its connection and leaving a small black mark on the circuit board.

My dad would simply look for the black mark and try to figure out which component was required to replace it. One two-cent resistor later, and he could resell that TV.

With computers, the concept was almost the same; however, instead of resistors, it was integrated circuit (IC) chips. Back then, the computers would often fail when one of these chips got too hot. So, he would identify the broken chip by using freeze spray to cool them, one at a time, until the computer booted up again. Then he'd replace the broken chip. This was the mindset that I was taught growing up. If something didn't work, we needed to figure out the problem ourselves. All it took was patience and logic.

When I was seven, I wanted to learn about computers, but we were well below the poverty line and could never afford one ourselves. This was in 1984, when the Apple II was still a top-of-the-line product. So, instead of buying one, we built our first computer using Steve Wozniak's design and the electronics lovers' community. At that point, even though a new computer was too expensive, every component we needed to create one could be found in local flea markets and swap meets. Once we had all the parts together, we mounted this "Apple" on a piece of plywood and called it a "banana" just to "think different."

By the time I was twelve, I had figured out the software part by installing a disk operating system, or DOS, and teaching myself basic programming. From there, I made my own *Zork*-inspired text-based adventure game. By the end of elementary school, I was a programmer who could assemble electronics.

I'd learned early on that our brains were our survival tools, and that night, tears drying on my face as I watched my dad perform another miracle using nothing but his wits and logic, I realized I was like the TV in front of him. My diagnosis meant that I was broken to some. I was given up on and labeled as flawed. But I still contained all the components to work perfectly. I just needed to get in there and fix it.

I started by taking the Exploding Keys Brainhack (page 19) technique further.

The Journey Brainhack

To remember where you placed your keys, you can imagine them exploding. But why stop at one item? We can expand on this idea to memorize many items—even hundreds.

Here is a list of random objects:

Thermometer	Rain
Statue	Tuning fork
Rock	Cereal
Chocolate bar	Dog
Juice	Butler
Chair	Mac and cheese

Many use repetition to memorize information, but often, repeating information over and over (rote memory) leads to recall that is full of errors and fades quickly. With practice, memory techniques can be nearly error free, fun, and quick, and can lead to understanding the material and not just being able to regurgitate it.

This particular method has a long history. Alternately called the "Roman room method," the "method of loci," or the "memory palace," emperors and kings used it to learn and remember everything needed to be a head of state.

To memorize a list in order, pick a room in your house or workplace that you are familiar with—a place you could close your eyes and visualize clearly. You will place these objects around your mental room in order, just like you did by visualizing the keys exploding.

I make rules about what direction I will mentally travel around the room. I go from top to bottom and left to right. This means if I have a light switch above a nightstand with a lamp and a clock on it, then a window beside it, the order of my list would be: light switch, lamp, clock, top drawer of the nightstand, under the nightstand, the curtain rod, window, windowsill, and so forth. This lets me take any room and make a linear list out of it. Here's an example using the list above and my room:

1. Imagine you stab the thermometer into the light switch and mercury drips down, causing sparks.
2. A Greek statue crushed the lamp.
3. The clock turns into a rock, still displaying the time.
4. There are a ton of melting chocolate bars in the top drawer, dripping down the nightstand.
5. You dropped your juice on the floor and it splashed under the nightstand.

Now you try . . .

Use a room in your house and do the same exercise, but make links that appeal to you.

Practice this on a few lists until it's second nature. Use it for to-do lists, studying, or just for staying sharp.

Oh, and the list I just gave you isn't a random list of objects, but actually the way I taught my son to recall the planets in the solar system.

Thermometer (Mercury)

Statue (Venus)

Rock (Earth)

Chocolate bar (Mars)

Juice (Jupiter)

Chair (Saturn—"Sat"-urn)

Rain (Uranus—Ur-"rain"-us)

Tuning fork (Neptune—Nep-"tune")

Cereal (Ceres, largest object in the asteroid belt, and a dwarf planet)

Dog (Pluto)

Butler (Haumea, pronounced how-may-ah—"How may I help you?")

Macaroni and cheese (Makemake, pronounced mak-ee mak-ee)

There is a "carry-on" effect when memorizing information with memory techniques rather than just repetition. Rote memory focuses only on the list or phrase we are repeating over and over to memorize and also fade quickly, but memory techniques give us more power by giving our brain a fuller picture. When you link information using these techniques, other details come along for the ride. For example, when you link a person's name to their face, you will start to recall other things too, like details of your conversations and other preferences they shared with you. This extra understanding comes from an interesting natural effect when stimulating your memory.

When you make a connection using visualization in the right way, you activate the reticular activating system (RAS). This opens up your brain's long-term memory, and in the process, other information comes along for the ride when you link it. You can be memorizing the names of generals in a war and, in the process, information like the battle's turning point gets connected too.

* * *

I decided that night to take charge of my brain and learn everything I could about how to hack it, leaving no stone unturned. I would search for real world hacks through books on memory, speed learning, speed-reading, neuroscience, and even mentalism, hypnosis, and much more. All along the way, I would experiment with what I learned, trying new ways to apply these techniques and even invent new ones. When I was ready, I would teach others.

CHAPTER **SUMMARY**

- When you want to remember items on a list, try the Journey Brain-hack to go beyond what is possible with rote memorization:
  - — **Step One:** Choose a room or series of rooms to use as your mental journey. Make sure you are already familiar with the layout of the room.
  - — **Step Two:** Go around the room from top to bottom, then left to right, linking an object to each location.
  - — **Step Three:** Review a couple of times just to make sure you didn't make a mistake.

5 | Pain Hack, Brainhack

The next day, I left for school late, riding recklessly and weaving my bike around, often against traffic. A horn sounded as tires screeched to a halt. I swerved, trying to avoid doing a discount Evel Knievel impression.

"Focus," I chanted to myself, ignoring my pounding heart.

Yes, it was my fault that I was late for school. For others, being late only meant two things: laziness and unreliability. My ADHD made me lose track of time or distracted me. But the worst thing about the morning was the pain. I have woken up each day with back pain for as far back as I can remember. So, jumping out of bed to race to school was impossible.

Anyone with chronic pain knows that there are good days and bad. On my good days, I could run and play with just as much zeal as my peers, but on bad days, I'd remember just how much of a cage my body was. Sometimes adults would use my good days as proof that I was faking my bad days.

That day on my bike was a bad day, so I packed a foldaway cane in my backpack just in case I needed it.

Not only was I late to school, I was also late to a meeting with the principal. Rushing into the main office, cane in hand, I saw a row of secretaries sitting along a long counter. Their constant chatter and shuffling of papers reminded me of crows on a powerline. Noticing I had come to the meeting without my parents, the paper mavens stopped their endless sorting of forms and looked up at me with a knowing expression. They'd seen me before. Their problem-kid radar was in full effect, and they knew I was going to be a regular visitor.

Being a fourteen-year-old kid walking with a cane had its pros and cons. Kids would make fun of me, of course, but they'd do it from a distance, as I did have a metal stick at my side. However, it was the adults' reactions that affected me the most.

"You're not allowed to bring that with you."

I looked up as one maven pointed at my cane.

"It can be used as a weapon," she continued.

"The only thing this fights is gravity," I joked, trying to lighten the mood. But the paper maven was ready to fight for her "just belief."

"I remember you from earlier, and you didn't need a cane to walk," she retorted, her voice raising with each word, "so stop faking for sympathy and hand it over!"

The noisy paper coop suddenly fell silent; everyone's eyes turned to the "problem kid" as they waited to see my next move. Sadly, I did the worst thing imaginable. I complied. As I surrendered my cane, my explanations of my pain's coming and going fell on deaf ears.

I decided to sit and escape into my imagination. They call it daydreaming, but it helped me. From the day I was born, doctors said I was going to die. I was hospitalized for the first eleven weeks of life, and I'm told the doctors were right. I did die twice. But the angels in uniform performed their miracles and brought me back.

I was in and out of the hospital for years dealing with chronic pain, sickness, breathing issues, and more. But the worst for me was the boredom. To stay sane as a child back in the hospital with nothing to entertain me but my thoughts, I would create elaborate stories and construct amazing machines in my mind.

At the time, I didn't realize I was using the principle of visualization. I was just trying to use my mind to stop my pain. My years of hospital boredom had been a training ground.

One trick I learned was how to fool my senses. I would stand up and put my feet together. Then I'd imagine I was on top of a building. I would ask myself questions and really sink deep into the image. Make it feel real; then mentally, walk to the edge and jump off. With practice, I got better and better until I felt a powerful reaction in my body as strong as riding a roller coaster and was able to feel the sensation of flying. Try it yourself.

Many brainhacks use visualization, but that word is about more than just the visual sense. When you imagine a hack, you should be using all of your senses to create a realistic scene in your mind's eye. I use the word *visualization,* but in reality, this process uses all your senses. I want to call it "sensualization," but that word sounds like it should be in a romance novel instead.

"The principal will see you now," the maven said in a monotone voice, handing me *the paper* that all my teachers had already seen.

"Student Dave Farrow shows signs of dyslexia, ADD, ADHD, and slow learning even with a high IQ. Medical concerns include dizzy spells, fatigue, and 'complaints' of chronic pain."

I remained seated, rereading the paper repeatedly. Yes, I'll admit that I did have difficulty focusing and could get distracted faster than a dog in a room full of squirrels. But I could learn quickly too. I just fell behind because of medical problems and couldn't figure out how to catch up. I also blanked out on tests, even when I really knew the information. The chronic pain was normal to me by now, though, so I had no idea how much it was hurting my grades.

As for the dyslexia, yes, I knew that letters did weird things when I read them too fast. It made spelling nearly impossible, but I still read well—just slowly. Then, I got really upset fixating on the word *complaints.* They'd put quotes around it. Did that imply it was fake? I had my medical records and doctors' notes. Why was it so hard to believe a kid had back pain?

BANG! The sound of a paper maven hitting the counter shook me out of my thoughts.

"I *said* the principal will see you now," she yelled.

I'd unintentionally hyperfocused on the page. *If only I could hyperfocus on my studies, I'd be superhuman,* I thought. I didn't realize it would be true one day.

Murphy must have been smiling because his law was in full effect; in that very moment, as I got up, a terrible pain shot from my back down my leg. I held back the tears, refusing to collapse and earn more words of discouragement from the mavens as I took one painful step at a time.

Ten painful jabs until I reach the chair in his office, I thought.

It was twelve.

As I entered Principal James's office, he gestured for me to sit and wait while he continued talking on the phone. That was good because I needed a few minutes to do another brainhack. It was a trick that I'd developed in the hospital while dealing with my chronic pain. As a child, I'd have bouts of pain and was medicated accordingly. One day, they stopped my meds out of fear of me developing an addiction.

The problem with pain is that it's invisible. You never know what someone is dealing with by looking from the outside. My pain led to depression, sleep problems, and poor academic performance. Addiction seemed equally horrible too, so I seemed to be stuck in a catch-22.

During those days, when the pain was unbearable and the only tool I had was my imagination, I developed a brainhack to push away the pain. Later in life, I taught this technique in my courses and freed people from years of pain. It was a combination of visualization and breathing. When done right, it allowed me to completely block out the sensation of pain. All I needed was a moment to concentrate.

Push Away Pain Brainhack

Millions of Americans suffer from migraines, joint pain, and fibromyalgia, and pain is considered the fifth vital sign in medicine—akin to one's heart rate and blood pressure. Pain is our body's way of telling us something is wrong, but what happens when the signal becomes the disease?

My process takes advantage of a natural visualization mechanism in the brain. In this way, we can change how our bodies perceive information, allowing us to mitigate pain. But like any tool, it can be used incorrectly. Follow these steps to get the most out of the Pain Hack.

Step One: Visualize the area in pain. Imagine every muscle, ligament, bone, organ, and/or nerve cell. Try to imagine it as clearly as possible, not in your mind's eye but as if you're looking through a scanner right into your body.

Step Two: Slow your breathing and become aware of your breath and blood flow. Try to get into a state of total awareness, focusing on the area in pain and blocking out any outside distractions.

Step Three: Let your body give you an image of the pain. Just be open to it; don't force it. Ask your body to show you what the pain looks like, and accept any visual representation it shows you. When I first tried this technique, I visualized my pain as rust-red-colored dust swirling around the pain point. But others have told me they see something else. The key is to imagine what your brain thinks the pain looks like; don't push your ideas onto it.

Step Four: Take deep breaths in, and as you exhale, imagine your breath is pushing on the pain. Watch the pain as it's slowly blown away by the wind your breath is causing. Don't rush or push too hard at first. Take your time, and let it happen over the course of several breaths.

This is similar to meditation, but it's unnecessary to take much time, go deep, or get into a trance. Just use your imagination. You should feel the pain lifting naturally.

There is one downside to this Pain Hack. To keep the pain away, you need to keep focusing. It doesn't require as much focus as it took to banish the pain in the first place, but if you want to keep the pain away, you need to keep visualizing your breath pushing at it, or it will return. I have used this technique many times to push powerful pain away in order to drift off to sleep—only for it to return at the last moment.

CHAPTER **SUMMARY**

- My Push Away Pain Brainhack is a visualization trick meant to fool the senses. All you need to do is imagine the area in pain; let your mind tell you what the pain looks like; breathe deeply and imagine the breath is a wind blowing at it; relax and let it go.

6 | Hack to the Future!

Back in the principal's office, with a few deep breaths, my pain was almost gone. As I looked up, I saw him staring at me.

"I was doing a thing to make my back feel better," I explained, embarrassed.

He just nodded at me, with no ridicule or judgment. I returned to the subject at hand, holding the paper up.

"What are my options?" I asked, still staring down at the paper in my hands.

Principal James hesitated for a moment before listing his plan. None of it sounded good. I would stay in general-level streaming, which were essentially boring topics that I hated. Then, I would spend a session every week in the resource room (a room filled with colors and games for those that needed "extra help"). That was it. It was as though I were watching a train wreck happen right before my eyes, and yet I could do nothing.

"Isn't there anything else I can do?" I pleaded. I knew that more challenges were really what I needed to focus.

With a heavy sigh, Principal James shook his head.

"Keep at the general level first. And if you get your grades up, then we'll definitely move you up." He smiled encouragingly, but the look in his eyes said it all. That would never happen.

As I tried to comprehend my fate, Principal James explained the education "streaming" (sometimes called "tracking") system. Kids were evaluated and then categorized as "general" or "advanced" before entering high school. The advanced-level kids were headed for college and university, and the general-level kids for something lower in status, like trades or minimum wage work. It basically recreates a class structure, instead of treating people as unique individuals.

The idea of sorting people based on aptitude isn't new. The factory system of learning was created to produce complacent workers and managers for the industrial revolution. If you think differently or challenge what the "accepted wisdom" is, you simply get even lower in status.

Whether it is general level versus advanced level, trades versus degrees, minimum wage workers versus executives, the bourgeois versus the proletariat, we tend to put people in boxes—for life.

Even today, I meet people who want to sort humans like cattle based on IQ, class, learning style, gender, race, political background, real-world experience, and other even crazier criteria. It's funny how the person doing the sorting always ends up near the top of their "unbiased" human sorting system. It reminds me of an episode of *Rick and Morty* where newly-created life-forms periodically launch out of a volcano into a machine designed to sort them by aptitude, creating the perfect society.

Spoiler alert: It did not end well.

Data tells us that individualization and cultivating multiple intelligences are the future of education. Success isn't a single bell curve but is determined by several different traits that depend on the type of task a person is performing. The same person who invents the next cancer cure isn't always the best person to get on stage and explain it to an audience.

For example, in multiple studies over several decades, the two traits that have proven most closely associated with financial success in life are self-confidence and grit (the ability to get back on the horse after failure). Unfortunately, though we can all acquire these traits with very little practice, no official time is spent on their development.

Listening to Principal James talk about educational streaming and my predetermined life, I wanted to escape back to my imagination. I had read something interesting about Winter Olympic athletes and how they would visualize every possible outcome of an event before it happened. For events like bobsledding and skiing, athletes often would get only a couple of chances to do a perfect run down a new track. So, they would visualize it over and over, imagining every twist and turn. This trained the body to believe the event had already happened, and their performance was incredible.

I wanted to do that with my life. I wanted to do a visualization of the twists and turns in my life that was so clear that it would help me succeed and prove all the critics wrong. I zoned out for a moment and started to visualize my possible future.

The more the principal talked about my diagnosis and its repercussions, the further my goals drifted. I felt like I was slipping out of my body. As I listened to the plans the school had made for me, as my mind wandered, I felt like my timeline was being split, allowing me to see the repercussions of this action ripple forward in time. Two possible paths became clear as I started to visualize the type of person I would be if I followed each path.

I imagined as clearly and unbiasedly as I could what person I would become if I followed each path. In the first path, I accept their plans for me with full compliance. I follow their advice, and the system labels me a "good boy" because I heed all their instructions while accepting my fate and lowering my ambitions. It's a tempting choice; I'd have a good excuse—a bogeyman of sorts—to point to and blame my problems on. No one would blame me for taking that path, and I could always say the "system" was failing me. Future me would be unhappy, but I would always have someone else to point the finger of blame at. A bitter shell of a man; sad and tired of living a life that could have been better if the system hadn't failed me.

I didn't like that man.

Then there was choice number two. It was fuzzy but nonetheless real: Become the potential person I wanted to be if I said no. If I just held fast

Future Visualization Brainhack

This visualization brainhack is the closest thing I have found to predicting the future. It's a way to make decisions and see their consequences with amazing accuracy before they happen.

Step One: Imagine the present situation. See it with all of your senses and make it real.

Step Two: Ask questions as you mentally travel forward in time. Things like: What will happen in ten years if I take this step? Keep an open mind and really be curious. Don't try to impose any opinion on the image. This takes practice.

Step Three: Remove personal bias. If the answer you get is too quick or something you know you are influencing, then try again. The key is to want the truth. It's easier to remove the bias when cultivating curiosity.

Step Four: Keep asking to see the consequences of different actions until your choice is clear.

---

to the belief that they were wrong about me, and I was right. I'd follow my own path, treating my brain like a broken TV I could fix. Even though I was just a fourteen-year-old kid at the time, I knew this was the right track. I was challenging hundreds if not thousands of certified, degree-holding teachers' and specialists' beliefs. But as crazy as it sounded, I knew I was right. I could make a difference and live the life I wanted to live.

I started to explain my thoughts to the principal. As I spoke, my excitement increased. I was in the zone. In my head, it was a turnaround worthy of a comic book origin story. The hero discovers a simple thing that gives him abilities beyond everyone else. What I would later call brainhacks. They were my secret power that would fix everything. It was so simple and straightforward. Then, I looked up.

Principal James was sitting there quietly as he listened to me, with an expression I'd seen so many times before. It was "the face" that a person made when they believed that you'd fail but didn't want to break the news to you. He showed a stoic calm, trying to hide the sadness of reality. Seeing "the face" made me realize that my life wasn't a comic book story, and it would never be easy. But I wasn't ready to give up.

"You keep trying," he said, with a forced smile and sad eyes. It was clear that he'd already given up, but he was kind enough to try to keep it to himself, so as to not crush my dreams. As we fell into silence, he hesitated for a moment. There was so much empathy in his eyes as he opened his mouth to speak, but holding my gaze for a few seconds longer, he closed his mouth and instead walked out of the room and returned with my cane. It was a kindness I'd never forget.

CHAPTER **SUMMARY**

- My Future Visualization Brainhack may seem simple, but what makes this different (and powerful) is that you are asking questions. Meditate and open your mind to possibilities. Get curious about what your future holds and ask your powerful brain what is likely to happen if you take each choice. You'll be glad you did.

AXIOM THREE

RARITY

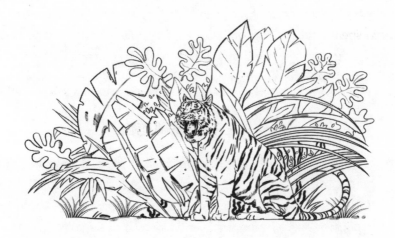

Imagine you're in the jungle, looking at the beautiful scenery. Going from left to right, you see the following: a rock, moss, a tree, a snail on a leaf, a small stream, another tree, a tiger, a big rock, two frogs on a . . . and now you're dead, because you didn't prioritize the tiger.

The brain focuses instantly on what is rare because that is where danger usually hides. The brain ranks everything in life based on how unique and uncommon it is, like antiques, precious metals, or collectors' items. The brain classifies "rare" as "valuable." It treats information the same way—and actually decides to focus on and remember it more. We can use this natural survival mechanism to trick the brain into permanently memorizing anything we want.

7 | The Memory Club

As I practiced the art of memory that year, everything started to make sense. I did much better on my end-of-year exams, and the next year, my performance in school had improved so much that my friends in the debate club noticed. One day, during a club meeting, some fellow students and two teachers, Mr. Muller and Mr. Simmons, asked about how memory hacks worked. Right then and there, I launched into a lesson. By the end of that class, I had the group recalling dozens of items forward and backward using the Journey Brainhack (page 24). This was the start of something great.

Mr. Simmons converted his debate club into what I was to find out later was the first high school club on memory techniques in the world. Today, there are memory clubs in schools around the world, and these techniques are even the subject of competitions. But at the time, it was completely new.

Week after week, my impromptu class grew, and even a few teachers attended. Then, someone walked in that I didn't expect to see.

"I wanted to see what you were doing here," Mr. Ross grunted, not sitting down.

I had just finished teaching the Journey Brainhack and showing my pupils how to create different journeys for different subjects.

"I've heard of this stuff before," interrupted Mr. Ross. "It's a kids' game to link objects in your head, but it doesn't work for most people."

"Actually, that's a perfect segue into my next point," I added, trying to take back control of the room. I had to remind myself that it was my club, not his geography classroom, and I didn't have to automatically defer to him. I started to describe the three reasons a memory link might not work and how to make it perfect. To do this, I used a metaphor.

THE TIGER IN THE JUNGLE

For most of human existence, our ability to recall information was related to our ability to find food and avoid danger, both of which involve noticing what stands out in front of us. If we see darker-colored ground, it could be wet from a water source; a broken tree could indicate a large predator pushed it over; and when noisy birds suddenly go quiet, it's a sign there is danger nearby.

The ability to notice what is novel helped us survive and evolve so much that a portion of our brain became dedicated to the task: the reticular activating system (RAS). It applies to everything we watch and hear, from education to entertainment to daily life. Think about it. Have you ever seen a movie about a guy who goes to work then comes home and watches TV? No, we like movies about action, suspense, or unlikely romance, because we find these things novel and thus interesting to the brain. Brain training takes advantage of this concept by using it to improve mental connections. A memory, for example, is just a connection between a question and the answer. Rarity is the glue that makes that connection strong. (Even the Exploding Keys Brainhack takes advantage of this—tying a location to a memorable, novel image.)

Countless times, people have come up to me at a seminar or corporate talk, explaining that memory techniques don't work for them, only for me to discover that they have been missing a few key insights. When linking information in your mind's eye, some links stick better than others.

After teaching these brainhacks to thousands of people, I discovered some hacks to help you achieve perfect memory links right away.

Mini Rarity Brainhacks

Here are three mini rarity hacks to make your memory recall perfect.

Stop, Drop, and Visualize

The most common reason a person forgets a link is distraction. Ask yourself: Did you stop your train of thought and imagine the sensory information in the image? For the technique to work, you need to stop paying attention to the external world and pay attention to only the internal world for a split second. Interestingly, this is the reason top-performing students find learning memory techniques hard—because they are not used to diving into their imaginations. The dreamers, artists, and rebels have the advantage here.

Practice Clarity

Many people aren't used to visualizing information. In fact, it's often discouraged. However, just having a good imagination or being creative isn't enough sometimes. It takes practice to clearly hold an image in your mind, but anyone can do it with time and patience, so keep trying.

Imagine Seeing Yourself

One way to improve your clarity is to imagine yourself in the image. Imagine either the event happening right in front of you as you reach out and touch it, or imagine seeing yourself from the outside, in third-person perspective. When people have difficulty with their image clarity, one of these two tricks will fix it.

Back in the memory club, I could tell I was making sense, and the room was interested. I could feel it. They were nodding and even taking notes, enthralled. But Mr. Ross couldn't hold in his annoyance anymore.

"This needs to end. You can't have a student teaching a teacher," he bellowed. "We need to maintain authority," he added, looking to the other teachers for support.

Mr. Muller, my mentor, replied with logic—the best remedy for bullies. "This is an after-school club, not a class. It doesn't damage your authority."

"David is acting like he knows more about learning than the entire education system," Mr. Ross rebutted.

I tried to step in to correct him that my techniques do not conflict with traditional learning. They're just an extra tool. But at this point, the two titans of education in my life had already squared off.

Mr. Simmons chimed in as well. "Mr. Ross, I believe you are a good teacher at heart. But we can all learn new things—and not just in the optional teaching credits you like to take. Memory is something we don't often talk about."

Ross tried to defend himself. "When I started out, I had wild ideas about transforming young minds too. I imagined my students on the news because they had done some amazing genius thing. But over the years, I have seen one simple truth. People don't change. C students can't just turn around and get the kind of test results he did"—he pointed at me—"by imagining some silly pictures."

He was referring to my recent turnaround in grades. When I started using memory hacks and stopped blanking out on tests, my scores didn't just get a small boost; on some tests, I more than tripled my grade.

"The key to life is to have reasonable goals and expectations, so you don't get disappointed. Never aim too high, or you will crash!" Mr. Ross continued.

Mr. Muller replied, "What happened to aiming high and inspiring kids?"

Mr. Ross sighed. "I'm trying to keep them from suffering—from believing in fairy tales that everyone has a genius inside them—only to be disappointed."

"Our job is to believe in these kids. Yes, it's disappointing when their reach exceeds their grasp, but that's the only way to know what their reach is. Then, we go back the next day and try again."

I swear, I heard an epic soundtrack behind his words. The conversation continued like that for a while until Mr. Ross left the room. It was then I realized that behind his harsh shell he actually thought he was doing the right thing.

CHAPTER **SUMMARY**

- Tiger in the Jungle: This is the principle that we have evolved to pay attention to things that stand out from the crowd. Knowing this, we can better understand how we interact with the world and what we remember.
- Stop Thinking and Visualize: The most common reason a person forgets a link is distraction. When you memorize something, stop your train of thought, and visualize the link as clearly as you can.
- Practice Clarity: People aren't used to visualizing information, so you will start with a faded image. Keep trying, and it will become clearer.
- Put Yourself in the Image: People who can't seem to visualize overcome it by putting themselves in the image, like imagining their own hand wrapping an item around the desk lamp in the Journey Brainhack. Imagining themselves in first person or third person works equally well.

8 | The Test

Like codependent lovers, success and failure have been the best of friends in my life. One seems to always want to follow the other. Almost as if they need each other.

The argument with Mr. Ross had an impact on me. So far, these brain-hacks had been fun and gave me confidence. They worked and raised my grades, but I never thought they could be a threat to the system. I would have laughed at the idea that imagining silly pictures could change other people's lives.

Now, by my second or third year of high school, I decided I wanted to do this for a living. I was going to push these hacks as far as they could go and make a business out of teaching them. The irony was that I only turned to brainhacks because of the educational system—because there was no instruction in *how* to learn.

Today, as a speaker, I travel to colleges to help students prepare for exams and improve performance. The story is the same in every college. First-generation college students have the toughest time getting higher grades. Not just because of the challenges that come from being mostly minorities from low-income families. After I teach my techniques, they come up to me, emotional, saying the same thing: that no one told them how to run their brain.

The basic brainhacks I'd learned so far had taken my performance from the bottom of all my classes to the upper middle within a few semesters. But it was just the tip of the iceberg. I had to get serious about my brainhacks. I had to make them even better.

I decided that it would be a good time to double down on brainhacks and try to get a perfect grade on a test. The ideal test was coming up in computer class. It was a test to remember computer commands. Some computer programs required the user to learn a list of key combinations to trigger commands instead of using a menu. Hit F9 to start spell check, or Shift+F6 to print, for example.

This test was ideal because it was a pure memory test with abstract items. Easy for someone with my techniques, but tough for everyone else. My strategy was to make an image for each command that linked the command to the right key using a special code for numbers and letters. (We will learn to use memory codes later in this book.)

I remember how much fun it was to think of the images and make the links. Time flew by, and it took only one evening to think of and memorize all fifty commands, with perfect recall.

In computer class a few days later, the teacher handed out the test. It took me only twenty minutes to fill in the answers and hand it in triumphantly. The look of surprise on the teacher's face made me smile, but in hindsight, I should have explained how I performed this feat.

He angrily checked the test against the answer key. As he marked every answer right, my smile got larger, but he wasn't smiling.

"I don't tolerate cheaters in my class, Mr. Farrow," he said.

"But I didn't cheat," I said. "I used memory techniques. Search me if you don't believe me."

"You can try to explain it any way you like, but it's not humanly possible for a student to get perfect on this test. Much less a student like you, David."

I knew what the last part meant. I got distracted and panicked on tests. No matter how much effort I put in, I would be the dumb kid, because that's what their expert assessed me as, and they believe their system more than their eyes. I didn't know what to do. I walked back to the desk with the paper in hand.

Then the teacher told me that I would have another chance to do the test in detention that night.

Watched over by Mr. Ross.

Great.

* * *

I was stopped trying to walk into detention.

"Remove your shoes," Mr. Ross ordered.

"Wait, what?" Surprised, I look around at other kids, and none of them had their shoes off.

"Remove your shoes. Those doodles could be code for the answers. It could be how you cheated," he said with a sly smile.

"So, I'm smart enough to figure out a secret code on these shoes that you can't decipher, but I'm not smart enough to just learn study techniques and do better on these tests."

"Don't be a smart ass, David!" he yelled. "It's not humanly possible to do that well on this test. Students don't go from bombing every test to scoring 100% overnight."

He wasn't holding back anymore. It was after school, and there were no other teachers around, so his volume was higher. I remember being surprised that his regular offensive teaching style was actually his version of good behavior.

"You're a stupid kid who thinks he's outsmarting people, but I see through it, and I *will* figure out how you're cheating. All these magic brain trick ideas you have are fake, and you will be exposed. Now sit down, and stop avoiding this test!"

I removed my shoes and placed them on his desk, realizing I couldn't talk sense to the man.

"Try not to forget your shoes when you leave," he said snidely.

I knew why he'd said that. As an ADHD kid it was common for my brain to hyperfocus or get distracted, making me prone to leaving stuff

Pattern Interrupt Brainhack

Most of us are walking around in a zombie-like state. We reenact patterns and get lost in our thoughts. I have made this into an art form. If you have ever left the water running or the stove on and forgotten about it, then you know how this feels. When we are in this state, we reenact old habits and patterns. The other day, I got in my car with the intention of driving to get groceries, only to start driving my office commute route until I "woke up."

We have all been there, and the solution is simple.

Place a physical object in your way that will break your pattern. This could be anything from a pen to a coffee cup. One student of mine was a warehouse delivery driver. He was under such pressure to complete his route fast, he kept forgetting to get signatures from his deliveries and was going to lose his job over it. The solution was to place a pen on his seat every time he left the truck. When he returned, he would have to move the pen to sit down and this broke his pattern, reminding him to get a signature.

You can take this to another level by adding a link to the interrupt. One night, when I was falling asleep, I suddenly remembered that I needed to call my accountant in the morning, or I was going to miss a deadline. I reached out for a retro Spider-Man figure I had sitting on my nightstand (yes, I have a Spider-Man figure beside my bed, because I'm a fun guy). I threw the figure on the floor between me and the door to interrupt my pattern in the morning. Then imagined Spider-Man throwing money around like he's making it rain. The next morning, I nearly stepped on Spider-Man and instantly remembered the accounting call.

behind when I left class, like my jacket or a book. Mr. Ross seemed to take pleasure in making fun of me when I did this, which only made me more stressed and likely to forget. I obviously wasn't going to forget my shoes, but my books were another story, so when I sat down, I placed my bookbag in front of me against my desk so I would have to move it to leave the room. I had gotten in the habit of doing this—it's what is called a pattern interrupt.

In detention, a copy of the computer codes test was handed to me while a few others got different make-up tests. Some didn't get a test—their punishment just involved sitting quietly. I got started answering the questions. They had been rearranged, but were essentially the same as they'd been before, and I had no trouble recalling the answers from the mental links I made earlier. When I finished, the clock said fifteen minutes had passed. I'd been even faster than the last time.

My feet were cold, and I was getting frustrated. But I knew if I handed in my test, I would be accused of cheating again, so I waited, mumbling to myself as my eyes and mind wandered around the room. My eyes landed on my shoes.

Staring at my shoes got me angry. I had figured out how to memorize information fast and easily and was called a cheater as a reward.

Mr. Ross looked up to see me staring at my shoes on his desk while clearly mumbling to myself as if reading them.

"Aha! David, I caught you," he exclaimed. "Keep your eyes on your paper."

That mistake led to two more weeks of doing all my tests in a separate room after class with my shoes off. I brought warm socks next time.

ESCAPE THE CRAB BUCKET

For me, the biggest challenge in helping a failing student to turn around their grades often wasn't explaining the brain techniques or transferring the skill. It was convincing others they had really changed.

Students who take my online course often need to say they have both a private tutor and an extra study group helping them in order to get teachers to believe their jump in grades is real.

Anyone who has tried to aim high finds the same thing happening. Even when you change, the mental image of you in others' minds does not.

If you want to lose weight, make money, travel, etc., it can threaten their idea of who they think you are and even how the world works.

There is a dark side to the Rarity Axiom. The RAS (reticular activating system) looks for what stands out in people as well as data. You can imagine the result. When you act differently around your friends, they notice. This can be good—like when you feel sick or depressed, they hopefully lend support. When you stand out from your peer group by attempting to reach higher on the social ladder, however, the RAS triggers, and often friends and family try to hold you back. This is the "crab bucket effect."

The crab bucket effect is a well-studied collectivist phenomenon in which groups of humans work to bring down those who try to reach higher levels within a given social hierarchy. It's named after the behavior of crabs in a commercial trap. Crab traps aren't really traps. They are simply cages with a hole at the top. Any crab that can fit in could also climb out. Trappers learned long ago, though, that leaving just one crab in the trap would prevent any other crabs from escaping. Instead of helping each other escape, they prevent it. The more crabs in the trap, the more claws reach up to undermine the attempts of that one brave crab that dreams of freedom. Call it envy, spite, or even good intentions . . . it is human nature to try and bring down people who want to rise above the group.

It was hard to understand Mr. Ross's irrational hatred of me at the time, or to keep from feeling angry about it. In detention, I was surrounded by people who were bitter or had given up . . . but as word spread about my brainhacks, things started to change.

Often, other students in detention would ask me how to memorize a piece of information. I remember one time a student leaned into me to ask how to memorize the cell cycle and the phases of mitosis. I told him to imagine his toe itching for mitosis (my-toes-itch). I then went through how to imagine links for the other parts; anaphase, for instance, became a *Star Trek* character named Anna with a phaser.

The Stoic Brainhack

The hack for this comes from the ancient Stoics, and even though we will focus here on the crab bucket, this hack will also solve a ton of interpersonal challenges in life, and even make you happier and more confident, if you practice it.

The stoics believed that all our suffering comes from the difference between our reality and our expectations, and the solution is to meditate to accept reality instead of focusing on why it's wrong or not fair.

If someone yells at you, instead of focusing on how wrong it is, Stoics would say you should accept that sometimes people are going to yell. If a person dies, Stoics would accept the loss rather than get angry. Even those wrongfully convicted of a crime would be encouraged to accept that the system is corrupt and try to make the most of it.

Before you get horrified by this, let me add that it was embraced by Nelson Mandela during his years of imprisonment. He said the Stoic philosophy helped him to be ready to heal his country instead of falling into bitterness and despair.

Stoics are famously calm and logical, so much so that Gene Roddenberry used them as the basis for Spock in the first *Star Trek* series.

In the case of a crab bucket situation, once you understand that people are evolved to react this way, you can use a Stoic attitude to accept it. If it is a friend who seems intent on holding you back, you can calmly sit them down and talk about how you want to reach another level in life, and you want their support. As for other people trying to bring you down, acceptance and Stoicism can keep you from wasting your energy on anger.

If the kid was someone I knew, I tried to make the link something that I thought would work for them, based on their interests. Feedback from another memory club meeting had taught me that though my techniques are good, my images do not work for everyone. Some students could not make the techniques work because my images weren't sticking in their minds. Eventually, I would realize that this is because memory links work best when they are tailored to the individual.

Memory Modes™

Teaching memory techniques over the years, I saw a pattern. I would give crowds of students examples of memory links to imagine, and while some had instant success, others struggled. I would tell an audience to imagine keys exploding and some would smile while a few simply could not do it. That's when I realized the RAS (that filtering system in the brain) has a personality. Over time, I experimented with teaching styles and discovered five different ways people liked to make links in the brain. These differences also indicated things like what movies and books people might like and even what careers they may enjoy. Just like today's streaming platforms use your preferences to better suggest new movies, I could improve their results by teaching to their memory style. Because there seem to be five modalities that people fall into based on what their RAS likes to focus on, I call these "Memory Modes."

This theory was the basis for our McGill neuroscience study, in which people who were using memory hacks performed three times higher when using the right memory mode. Interestingly, these modes can also predict what entertainment and jobs you will enjoy.

Here are the modes:

1. Action: Likes sports and action movies; descended from the spirit of the clan's hunter. The best links for this mode involve movement.

2. Exaggeration: Likes the extreme versions of things; always looking for the next level. When learning a history lesson, for example, those in this category will recall the fine details of a battle better if they imagine thousands of soldiers in the field.

3. Oddity: Likes puzzles, sci-fi, and is the detective of a group; correlates to a career in science.

4. Personal: Focuses on how information relates to them. This mode correlates to careers like politics, acting, or sales.

5. Fantastical: The magical brings these minds to life. Bored by the ordinary world, they are dreamers who imagine possibilities that don't exist yet. Likes art and fantasy.

Here's how the different modes would most effectively connect an item like keys to a location in the Exploding Keys Hack.

Action: Focus on movement—make the keys explode.

Exaggeration: Make items numerous or bigger—imagine millions of keys or one giant key in the location.

Oddity: Focus on switching items to make odd combinations, like making the table made out of keys.

Personal: Focus on things connected to themselves—imagine the keys glued to their hand in the location.

Fantastical: Focus on the impossible, like the keys coming to life and talking.

Many have a combination of modes, and an exact test is available on our site, www.memorymodes.com.

Somehow, I had turned the punishment of two weeks' detention into a marketing opportunity. A few weeks later, my debate-turned-memory club was packed—standing room only.

CHAPTER **SUMMARY**

- To use the Pattern Interrupt Brainhack, put a small item in your way that will break your pattern to remind you of important things. Add a memory link to make it more powerful. Absentmindedness is a function of attention. The pattern interrupt uses your RAS to wake your brain up. It causes you to pay attention to what's important and breaks you out of the walking trance.

- The dark side of the rarity axiom and RAS means that we pay negative attention to people who stand out from the crowd. Troublemakers, ideological rivals, or people in our own group who are trying to make a better life can become targets. Like crabs in a bucket, other people can sometimes try to keep you down. To hack the crab bucket, sit down with these people to continuously change their mind or be willing to let them go. Be aware and keep climbing.

- To use the Stoic Brainhack, no matter what happens, accept that it is normal. Bad things happen to good people, and if you want the strength to fight it, getting upset will not help. Accept reality for what it is, be happy, and then seek to change it from there.

- Memory links work best when they are customized; use Memory Modes to find what will work for you. While most personality tests are little better than astrology, Memory Modes theory came from data involving thousands of people learning in live events. The conclusions of this theory were then supported by a double-blind study. People tend to fit into five different categories based on what their RAS focuses on most. These can correspond to the ideal way to imagine a memory link as well as things like entertainment preferences and career interests.

BRAIN PLASTICITY VS. HARDWIRED BRAIN

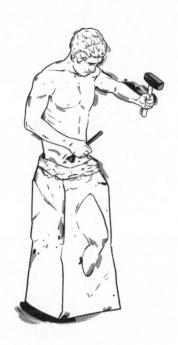

There has been a revolution in neuroscience. Today, we know that the brain is plastic (changing). With the right stimulation, you can heal, train, and change areas of the brain. Until recently, though, the scientific consensus was that the brain did not change or grow after puberty. It took a superman doing the impossible to get science to believe in change again.

9 | Go Hack Yourself

Morty: I can't change my nature.

Rick: Everyone can change their nature, Morty. It's what defines our species. Look at Iron Man. That actor was an animal in the '90s, literally waking up in bushes. His agent had to catch him with a butterfly net.

—*Rick and Morty*, **"Rickdependence Spray"**

So, nerve cells are different from other cells?" I asked the neurologist during a medical check-up.

If you have chronic pain, at some point, you meet a neurologist. It sparked my curiosity about the brain, and I was asking him a series of questions about how to get smarter.

"When we put them under a microscope, all other cells in the body divide when stimulated, but a nerve cell doesn't. Instead, it does grow connections," the doctor explained. "So, experts think you only have so many nerve cells, and when they die, you can't get more. That includes your brain."

"Yeah, I've seen the 'Just Say No' PSAs on drugs. They say every day cells die, and you can't get those cells back. But that would imply that no one can substantially improve their brain after puberty," I said, realizing that Mr. Ross's theory was backed up by the science of the day. "What about people who recover from head injuries or stroke?" I asked, recalling the experience of an uncle of mine. "You can train the body and brain over time to get better at any skill. That would grow new cells, right?"

"You don't get new cells. You just add more connections to the ones you have, and in those cases, we believe that the body was functioning less well but wasn't as injured as first expected, and after some time, it was able to return to normal. Like when a bruise's swelling goes down," he replied, enjoying the questions.

Even though that sounded like a work-around, I wanted to know more.

"What about pain, though? I feel pain that doesn't correspond to a physical injury. You can't see it on an X-ray. That doesn't mean I'm not hurt. Just that you can't see what is damaged," I concluded.

"One problem happening here is that nerves are being overactive and sending false signals of pain," he explained. "We have seen recovery from pain without any detectable physical change."

I was very aware of the idea of "false" pain. My mother suffered for years looking for the cause of her pain, and eventually she was just sent to psychiatrists rather than specialists.

Today, they would call this gaslighting.

I thought for a second. Something seemed off. The explanation didn't match experiences my family and I had seen.

"So, there are two possibilities then," I summarized. "One is that there is phantom pain—false signals—plus nerves that *seem* to repair themselves, but are really just turning back on after swelling goes down. But, at the same time, some nerves are overactive, sending extra signals that you have no way to measure or detect or even prove exist." I smiled, making a connection.

"Or option two: there is damage, an injury, or something cellular that's causing pain that you can't detect, and the body does have a way to repair nerve cells that we haven't discovered yet. Right?"

Instead of being annoyed, he paused for a minute, and then he told me of another theory.

THE THEORY OF BRAIN PLASTICITY

The scientific consensus at the time was the hardwired brain theory: the idea that nerves were static and didn't grow, which 99% of the research on the brain at the time had concluded. It was established science . . . and it was wrong.

That day, the doctor told me of a fringe group of scientists who believed the brain could change and recover from injuries. They gathered thousands of stories of miraculous recoveries from nerve injury. If true, this theory would mean that we can stimulate the brain into getting smarter or learning faster. The theory is called brain plasticity. It's a theory that your brain and nerves grow, repair, and rewire themselves as time goes on, and if true, it meant I could hack my brain. Even though the scientists thought the matter was settled, what I was learning contradicted their mainstream theory.

And it wasn't just me—the art of memory training has a two-thousand-year history dating back to ancient Greece. Some philosophers were famous for memorizing thousands of pieces of information in a public square. It was said that Aristotle's students learned memory training as one of their first subjects. Alexander the Great and Napoleon used these tools to recall names and details of every person in their armies, too. Memory training was even used in ancient Rome and China as well, to give emperors and elites an edge, and even today, there is a group of monks in northern India that use this same art to memorize long lists of words as part of a meditation technique. Throughout that rich history, memory training was tested time and again in the real world. Contrary to hardwired brain theory, my studies showed me that the brain could change and even achieve genius levels at any age.

The doctor's next words broke me out of my trance. "But no one takes that theory seriously," he said.

"Well," I said, quoting something I'd heard on TV, "no one took Einstein seriously at first either! After that, every great human advancement started as heresy."

Thousands of studies at the time confirmed this hardwired brain theory. But I believe they only confirmed what people already believed. Today, that theory has been abandoned, but many people still believe in the spirit behind it. They believe that we cannot change our habits, intelligence, or learning speed. This bias holds back so many.

Sometimes, we have faith in science without critically thinking for ourselves, and we run the risk of pushing bad science as a result. That's what happened with the hardwired brain theory. I talk to people who think it's offensive to encourage people to change, set goals, or think positively. What I call self-help or personal growth, others call toxic and blaming the individual.

What they don't understand is that change begins at home. When facing challenges, the best strategy in life is to try to affect them yourself first, and then change the world from a place of strength. Blaming society or circumstances feels good in the short term. To me, though, it's akin to giving up on the *potential* of an individual, and that is the most offensive thing I can imagine.

I used to grind my teeth. It's a bad habit born of boredom and fidgeting. When I got stressed, I did it to the point of getting headaches. This was a perfect example of brain plasticity at work. At first it was fun. Tapping my teeth, tapping my teeth together to the beat of a tune . . . over time I stopped noticing it and would grind them past each other till they ached.

It was time to use brain plasticity to end this habit. The first step to making a change is to become aware of it. In fact, simply being aware of how often you perform the action is extremely powerful. The simplest mindfulness brainhack is just to start counting.

Pick a small annoying habit you want to change—anything from subconscious eating or saying "um" too often to major compulsions. Start by simply counting the number of times it happens.

I knew if I just counted in my head that it would be easy to lose track, so I carried around a small piece of paper and a pen. This was essential, because keeping track outside of your head makes it more real. Like writing down your goals, it means more.

Activate Brain Plasticity Hack

Not only can the brain change, but it is also always changing based on what we habitually do.

Step One: Be aware of what you want to change first. Most of us aren't aware of how many negative thoughts and limiting beliefs we have.

Step Two: Take on a challenge. The greatest amounts of plasticity come from learning new things. For example, if you play crossword puzzles every day, you're only playing a game, but try brushing your teeth with the wrong hand, and now your brain is working hard.

Step Three: Make a routine and keep going. The brain does change, but it resists the process initially. Keep at it. Try building new habits every day for thirty days at least.

At first, I didn't write down any tics because I was doing it subconsciously. Then, on the second day, I caught myself twice after I had been grinding for a few minutes. So, there were two tics on the sheet.

On the third day, I counted over forty times that I tapped and ground. It's not uncommon to be surprised by how extensive your habit really is. After all, it's subconscious. Sometimes, I would be dreaming and grind my teeth in the dream and mark it down . . . only to wake up and wonder if a dream grind should count.

I kept going. Becoming more and more aware over the next two days, I had forty-five tics and peaked at sixty. Then, the number started to go down. At first, I would notice after I had ground my teeth and stop sooner than usual. The headache went away. Then, after a couple of days, I would notice when I was about to grind my teeth. The number went down quickly after that, from thirty-five to twenty to four. I still had the urge to grind them thirty-five times a day but stopped myself each time. For a few days, I had no tics but still felt the urge. But I had to stop myself less and less often until the urges stopped altogether.

The Counting Hack

Counting is the simplest way to be aware of your habits. It works for a while, but keep in mind that habits can come back if you don't pay attention. I needed to do the counting hack several times before I really got a handle on it.

Here it is step by step:

Step One: Make a rule about what you will count. If you're eliminating negative thoughts, do you count minor complaints about life or just thoughts directed at yourself?

Step Two: Use an external tool to count, like a note on your phone or a paper record. Somewhere you can see the progress. I like to mark it down on paper so it's permanent.

Step Three: Start trying to count. I say try because at first you will miss it happening or realize it happened afterward. That's fine. Just count it and move on.

Step Four: Total a number for each day and keep counting until the number goes down. Change happens over time, so be patient.

I was told by some friends who study the brain that the counting hack can disrupt drug trials and behavioral neuroscience studies. For example, I was told about a study about changing negative thinking that compared a drug to behavioral therapy. But to study that, the scientists would need a baseline. Just how many negative thoughts do people have in a day? So, of course, the groups were asked to count them.

Like many studies, there was a control group, a drug group, and a third assigned to some behavioral action like writing in a journal or watching a comedy show. The people taking the drug lowered their negative thoughts, but so did the group doing the behavioral tool. But the surprise was that the control group reduced just as much. Just counting and reporting the number of times they had negative thoughts reduced them. Awareness brings about change.

CHAPTER **SUMMARY**

- The belief that we cannot change our habits, intelligence, or learning speed is a bias that holds many back.
- You can Activate Brain Plasticity by being aware of what you want to change, taking on a challenge, and making a routine until your change is habit.
- If you want to stop a bad habit, count it away with the Counting Hack.

10 | Believe in Change

History has shown us what horrors unfold when society abandons the idea of self-improvement.

Leaders in the '90s and 2000s used the hardwired brain theory (HWB theory) to justify terrible policies that continue to hurt society today.

Bill Clinton's administration cited hardwired brain science in several criminal law reforms, like large mandatory minimum sentences, the three-strikes law (which locked people up and threw away the key after they committed three crimes), and more. This contributed to the modern prison industrial complex, where today America imprisons more people per capita than any other nation—most of whom are minorities. This is what happens when a society gives up on individual change.

Around that time, Hillary Clinton coined the term "superpredator" to talk about (predominantly Black) career criminals that the science claimed were hardwired to be violent. It was a phrase that would return to haunt her in her 2016 presidential run.

Every '90s drug PSA shows how drugs kill brain cells that will never grow back (based on HWB theory). Since reform and recovery was considered unscientific, funding moved from addiction support to a war on drugs—driving narcotics pricing up and creating a cartel boom. The more the United States fought drugs, the more power they gave them.

This is the difference between a fixed and a growth mindset. It's easy to get into a rut in our lives or think that we can never change because of our DNA or past circumstances, but history tells us the danger this thinking can lead to.

Early in my career I toured TV and radio stations, giving interviews as "the memory guy." I did over two thousand interviews in the late '90s to early 2000s, and this was my most controversial point. When I told everyone that the brain can change, doctors and scientists called me irresponsible for pushing fake science. Have you ever felt like the whole world was wrong and you were right? I'm happy to say the science is against them now.

Growth Mindset Hack

Follow these steps to switch to a growth mindset.

Step One: Be aware. Ask yourself questions about what you really believe. It may surprise you that the goal you've been working toward for months is something that you really don't believe can happen.

Step Two: Mentally zoom out from your specific situation. Something at work might seem really important, but it seems like a speck of dust after you zoom out. Also, realize that everyone gets a string of bad luck. Just being aware of the fixed mindset can often stop its progress.

Step Three: Think about others who have achieved your goal. Think about others who have been in your situation and gotten out of it. For every terrible tragedy, there's an inspirational story. If they can do it, so can you.

That's why it's important to cultivate a growth mindset in ourselves and the next generation. The person who changed it all had the ultimate growth mindset . . . Superman.

THE SUPER BRAINHACKER

Christopher Reeve was known for playing Superman. Later in life, a freak accident—being bucked off a horse—broke his spine, making him a person with quadriplegia. Doctors told him his nerve cells couldn't repair themselves, but he refused to give up. Every day, he would be suspended in a pool as volunteers moved his legs while he visualized the same movement in his mind's eye.

Habit Trigger Hack

The Counting Hack works to break bad habits, but they will come back if not replaced with good habits.

Habits have three components.

The trigger: This is what initiates the habit. It could be an alarm clock that starts a morning routine or a TV show that triggers us to start snacking. If you are thinking your bad habit just comes out of nowhere, one of the most common triggers is boredom.

The action: This is the habit itself. It helps to break this down into steps, but it has to be one overall activity. Snacking, for example, includes preparing the snack right before but does not include buying it in the store.

The reward: This is what you are getting out of the habit, like a feeling of being full or just satisfaction.

Create new habits by figuring out all these components first.

Step One: Use the same counting method from the Counting Hack on page 64 to break your habit while creating a new one. Keep track of every time you have a trigger. If it's TV watching, count the number of times you binge-watch per week.

Step Two: For each trigger, go through the motions of your positive habit. Make it as simple as possible. The key is that if you need to think while doing it, then it's not a habit—it will never become subconscious. Your habit can have multiple steps, but the biggest mistake people make is to make it too complex. Getting up to jog is easier than getting up to do a complex series of circuit training exercises.

Step Three: Finally, make sure you get a reward for doing this habit. Even a simple moment of looking in the mirror congratulating yourself can work wonders. Make it part of the habit, and if you are replacing a bad habit, make sure the new habit has a reward that is just as good as the bad habit.

One interesting way I used this was to take others' negative comments to cue me to think of positive ones. Growing up, everyone with ADHD hears lots of negative comments. Every time I heard a statistic or a dig about how a high percentage of ADHD people fail, I would tell myself that I was in the smaller percentage that overperformed. This became subconscious eventually, and I don't think I would have had the confidence to attempt a Guinness record without it.

Then after years of this effort, miraculously, his toes could move, and he could feel parts of his legs. The impossible was now possible, and scientists rushed to study him. This led to the discovery of pockets of naturally occurring stem cells in the spinal cord and brain stem. The body seems to be able to create an endless supply of them specifically to repair nerve cell damage. One person with a growth mindset changed science and society along with it. Imagine what you could do.

The first step to a growth mindset and embracing brain plasticity is to look at your habits. Changing a habit seems difficult, but it can be done.

CHAPTER **SUMMARY**

- Fixed vs. Growth Mindset: We can choose to look at life as fixed and limited. That all that is wrong cannot change. Or we can look at life as growing and reaching new levels and over time improving in big and small ways. The data supports the second view.

- Using the Habit Trigger Hack, you can replace bad habits and form new ones by figuring out the components of the trigger; counting each trigger and trying to perform new actions; and getting the reward each time, as long as the new habit makes the reward as good as what it's replacing.

THE SPEED OF THOUGHT IS RELATIVE

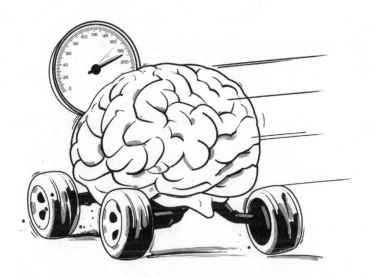

The brain measures information by comparing it to something else. Everything from temperature, reading speed, and even how spicy food tastes is all relative to the last time your brain experienced that sensory input. This is why quick changes are felt strongly—like going from a hot room to a cold one. But change slowly, and you can get used to almost anything.

Speed-reading takes advantage of this axiom with exercises that speed up the brain's points of comparison and thus can change reading and thinking speed.

11 | Speed-Reading, First Steps

The resource room was well lit with round tables and fun-looking areas. It was a catch-all place for people needing extra help—for those with everything from autism to language-learning difficulties to, of course, ADHD and dyslexia like me. I was here for a meeting with Mr. Lake.

Mr. Lake was looking at my diagnosis sheet and making comments. "Mr. Ross says you aren't engaging in the lessons," he stated, but paused as if it were a question.

I wanted to say his class was more like a low-budget Stanford prison experiment than a lesson to engage in. Fumbling, I replied, "I already know that stuff. There was no challenge."

He frowned at me. He was either a terrible actor or simply unwilling to hear me out. "Why ask me a question if you think I'm a liar?" I said . . . in my mind . . . to myself . . . like a coward.

This man was here to help me with my learning disabilities, but it didn't start off on the right track.

"I'm good at learning on my own," I said, looking to turn this around. "When I was nine, my dad and I built an Apple II computer from flea market parts." Aiming to impress, I doubled down. "I taught myself how to program it in BASIC. So, I know I can learn if I put my mind to it."

"Well . . . being at a basic level in computers is nice," he replied, half listening.

"No. BASIC is a programming language," I protested, then trailed off. "It's actually pretty advanced . . . never mind."

To address my dyslexia, Mr. Lake gave me a device that was supposed to help me read. It was a blue plastic board to lay atop a book page, with a white bar automatically moving down the page, supposedly to guide the eyes. As it moved, it made a loud sound reminiscent of the old game *Perfection*. I half-expected something to pop out when the bar got to the bottom.

How to Calculate Reading Speed

Reading speed can change by topic and genre. Knowing your reading speed helps identify any reading issues, and it's the first step to reading faster. Reading speed is calculated in words per minute, or WPM. To discover your reading speed:

Step One: Time yourself reading for ten minutes at a pace that will give you full comprehension. Not skimming or rushing.

Step Two: Count the number of lines you read and multiply that by the average number of words per line (AWPL).

Step Three: Divide by the number of minutes you read.

We use the average words per line because it would be crazy to count each and every word. Just count the number of words in a few sample lines and average them out. If you see a mix of six-, seven-, and eight-word lines, then pick seven as the average.

Formula for Reading Speed:

WPM = (# Lines × AWPL) ÷ # Minutes Reading

I tried using it for a while, but the bar actually made it more difficult to read, as it was never timed right, often blocking words mid-sentence or making me wait around for the next line to show. But the worst part was the distracting noise. I gave it a strong effort for weeks, and my reading comprehension and speed actually went down. I know this because I started learning about speed-reading around the same time, and the first step in the process was to be able to calculate my reading speed.

A quick note to readers: In this chapter, each brainhack is a part of the larger process of learning to speed-read.

My passion for speed reading would eventually lead me to work with Howard Berg, the world's fastest reader (and now my close friend too), and to be hired by Sony as a spokesperson for reading and education. But like many good things, it started with frustration. I started to search every resource I could find on speed-reading and dyslexia in my first few years in high school.

The most important thing is that reading speed needs to be improved in stages. If you skip a step, it can be difficult to get results. Start with this hack below and follow along up through Chapter Thirteen.

Subvocalization

A small percentage of readers move their tongue and lips almost imperceptibly while they read. Subvocalizing is a leftover from early in our reading development, when we sounded out words, but unfortunately, it keeps you reading slowly.

To test if you subvocalize, try holding a pen in your top lip by curling it up against your nose while you read. This uncomfortable position is so delicate that any attempt to subvocalize will make the pen drop.

Read this way for a chapter to make sure the pen does not move. If it does, keep practicing with it on your lip, noticing when it moves. This becomes a type of feedback system to teach your brain to stop subvocalizing. When you are ready, it's time for hand-eye coordination.

CHAPTER **SUMMARY**

- Before you can speed-read, you need to measure your reading speed. Time yourself for a few minutes reading at a steady pace with full comprehension. Then, take the number of lines you read and multiply that by the average number of words per line, and divide by the number of minutes to find your speed. Note: Reading speed can vary depending on the material.

- Subvocalization is the subconscious act of moving lips while reading. A high percentage of adults subvocalize as they read and do not even know it. To test whether you do, and whether you need to fix it, try holding a pencil between your upper lip and nose while you read. If it moves, then you are subvocalizing.

12 | Eye Guides

Frustrated with the blue board, I asked Mr. Lake questions. "Why does the bar move down? I've learned that reading-eye training should go back and forth like a pendulum instead to train my eyes to read better."

"Your eyes don't need training, and you should have outgrown the need for a finger to guide your eyes to read years ago," he rebutted. "This is designed to help you focus your ADHD and dyslexic brain on a smaller part of the page at a time," he explained holding up the blue board.

The truth is our eyes never grow out of the difficulty of moving in a straight line. This is because eyes aren't biologically good at going back and forth like a typewriter. I sighed. "Our eyes are balls in a socket, not sitting on rails."

I continued. "Here's a great way to demonstrate how our eyes work: Hold your arm up in front of you, as if you are saying stop. Lock your elbow, and try waving your arm left and right quickly. After thirty seconds, your shoulder will feel tired because it's a ball in a socket joint. Just like your eyes."

I went to the board to explain my point by drawing a picture of an eye with small muscles pulling on it. "As we read, the muscles in the eye start to strain because our eyes fight these movements. It's not natural."

I concluded, "This shaky movement instinct is a survival mechanism to protect us from predators by allowing the eye to catch movement."

"The only predator in this school is your upcoming test," Mr. Lake joked, "Seriously, though, haven't our eyes just gotten used to this movement?" he said, beginning to get interested.

I told him that training the eye does work somewhat, but most people's eyes still fight the movement, and it leads to eye strain. That's why people who read a lot often need glasses later in life.

"The solution is to use your finger, to train the eyes and brain to coordinate," I continued.

"But you're a grown-up person; you shouldn't still need your finger to help you read like kids do," he replied.

"No, not to help me read—to help me speed-read. Really fast," I replied with a smile, loving every minute of this now. "Speed-readers use their fingers to read—not as training wheels but as a power boost."

GIVE READING THE FINGER

The reason this works is that our eyes love to follow movement—like a dog chasing a ball. Just walk down the street, and every few seconds some movement will catch your eye. It could be a car driving to your left or a bird flying above you. Anything that moves, our eyes catch it and instantly go into action looking right at it.

You will never get eye strain following the movement of birds or a tennis match even though your eyes go back and forth repeatedly because the natural tendency of your eyes is to follow movement. When there is movement, then the muscles don't fight each other, and I find there is no strain. (If you are concerned about eye strain, consult your optometrist—your mileage may vary.)

"I don't believe it. Using your finger to read is going backward," Mr. Lake said, walking over to a shelf to pick up a book and handing it to me. "If you can read faster this way, then show me."

The Hand Guide Hack

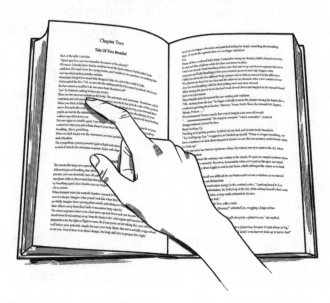

Step One: Use your hand to guide your eye across the page. Experiment with different hand positions, like using your pointer finger to aim at the words or using your palm to reveal them. Either way, the goal is to focus on the words, not your hand. Point at the words you want to read.

Step Two: Practice. This will feel weird at first and lower your comprehension because a hand on the page distracts you. Keep going until you're comfortable before trying to read faster. You may also notice smoother reading without getting "stuck on words." When you read without your hand as a guide, your eye gets stuck from time to time. I've noticed that, for me, straight up-and-down letters like L and I tended to be the ones that tripped me up. But with the hand to guide me, I didn't get stuck.

Just then, I noticed the small crowd that had formed around me. Others in the room had stopped to listen to our conversation, and even a few people walking by joined us. I grabbed the book and sat down with a deep breath and held the book open with my right hand while waving my hand across the words with my left.

At first, I went slowly and heard a chuckle, so I increased to my regular practice speed. Then, even faster. My hand fluttered down page after page. Ten pages later, he grabbed the book from my hands and then tested me on the contents. I answered his questions correctly.

Getting upset, Mr. Lake said, "You must have read this before. There is no way a person with dyslexia can read this fast."

* * *

Many students have come to me over the years asking about dyslexia, but it's a wide spectrum. Different people have more or less extreme versions of the same condition. My dyslexia is considered mild and becomes more prominent when I become stressed or try to rush through a task. Speed-reading changed all that for me. But you may be different. Dyslexia has several versions, from surface dyslexia (taking longer to process reading material and decode letters) to visual dyslexia (issues with visual sequencing in reading) to dyscalculia (reordering numbers).

I had a little of all of these, and I even reversed the 7 and the Jack when memorizing playing cards because they rotated in my mind to look alike. And like many dyslexics, my spelling is atrocious. (Yes, I had to look up how to spell the word "atrocious" just now.)

Most of the theories I encountered in the resource room were useless and based on some expert educator who wrote a book or made up a syllabus with little to no objective data that it worked.

One hack from the book *The Gift of Dyslexia* helped me. The exercise involves pulling your head back from the page and increasing your field of vision. But the biggest improvement came when I learned to speed-read. It may sound strange, but to me, normal slow reading was difficult. Speed-reading exercises actually made it easier, mainly because they

trained my eyes to read words in blocks or chunks by sight without sounding them out, and thus reversing a few letters here and there didn't hurt my
ability to read the words.

CHAPTER **SUMMARY**

- Though we don't usually think of it this way, our eyes are a ball in a
  socket pulled on by small muscles. Like other socket joints, the eye
  does not like to move back and forth in the same direction. It resists
  this movement—it's designed to catch the movement of predators
  in the wild, not to move horizontally across a page. However, when
  we give the eye movement to focus on, it follows it smoothly, making reading easier, healthier, and faster.

13 | The Wartime Technology of Speed-Reading

World War I was a horrible mess of trench warfare. Each side was dug in, making progress impossible. However, a new technology called the airplane was changing things. At first, planes were used to spy, then drop small bombs. Finally, it became clear that one plane could be used to shoot another plane out of the air, and the age of fighter planes was born. These planes looked nothing like modern Air Force marvels. They were made of balsa wood, wrapped in fabric, and held together with glue and willpower. The engines were weak too (by today's standards). They made these planes slow-moving and slow-turning.

The difference between living and dying lay in the skill of the pilot. Some tactics like attacking the enemy from above with the sun to your back—using gravity and blinding light to your advantage—made a difference. Many pilots, like the Red Baron fighting for the Central Powers, became famous destroying other planes using special tactics.

To fight back, the Allies took a survey of pilot experiences. They discovered that other than initial position, the biggest factor in deciding who won the dog fight was quick sight. The first pilot to see the other and react by moving their (slow) plane toward them set themselves up for success and was almost guaranteed to win the dog fight.

The air force got to work on strategies to improve reaction time and visual recognition. Interestingly, they were trying to train young people in skills that parents try to avoid today, because they usually come after hours of video game practice.

To help training, they created a large device the size of a refrigerator that would flip pictures past pilots at different speeds. The hundreds of pictures would depict things they would see while flying, like trees, lakes, clouds, and other planes. When they saw another plane, they were supposed to hit a button.

Information is scarce on this project, so it's not clear if this training device made a difference in the war effort. But one thing never changes. People get bored at work. One night, the technicians decided to replace the pictures of planes with words and flip them past each other to see what would happen. After a period of adjustment, they started to recognize the words without having to sound them out. This effect lasted beyond the training time and stayed with them for the rest of the day and week. With more practice, people said they were able to read like the wind.

This was the first known example of real natural sight-reading— the ability to recognize and understand some words without sound just because the word was flipped past them far faster than they could read. I like the idea that when I speed-read, I'm following a sort of accidental tradition that can trace its origin back to those brave men who flew back then.

IT'S ALL RELATIVE

Ever hear about the frog test? The idea is that putting a frog in boiling water will make it jump out. But if you place it in warm water and raise it to a boil slowly, it will not move. I always wondered where these morbid sayings came from. Like "killing two birds with one stone" and "there's more than one way to skin a cat." The past is brimming with dark humor. The frog story may not be technically true, but it is based on a real principle of the nervous system. We don't measure any data objectively. We only compare it to the last measurement.

To see this phenomenon in action, place your right hand in cold water for thirty seconds; then, put both hands in warm water. The right hand will feel much hotter. This is because experiences of hot and cold are relative only to the last thing that the sensor felt.

Baseball players use this principle to hit harder too. Before going up to the plate, every player grabs a bat with a weight on the end and swings it a

---

Overclocking Your Brain

After you are comfortable reading with your finger guiding you, take it to the next level.

Step One: Read in short three-minute bursts while following your finger across the words three to five times faster than you are comfortable with. You're not speed-reading yet, because you won't likely understand anything you attempt to read this fast. But your brain doesn't know that. Your brain just thinks this is the new normal it needs to adjust to. Think of it like simulated reading; don't zone out or blur your eyes. Instead, give it a real try to read all the words—just far faster than you can really comprehend.

Step Two: After a few timed intervals and breaks, you'll notice that you're picking words out here and there. Bits and pieces are made aware to you. This is your brain adjusting to the new speed. Now you're ready to test your speed again. Go to a new spot in the book that you haven't read or skimmed, and try another reading speed test. Read as fast as you comfortably can without losing comprehension. It can take time to find the sweet spot, but you should see your natural reading speed grow—and even double and triple—over time.

As for spelling? These days, everyone seems to have lost the ability to spell, and every device has spell-check, so even a dyslexic ADHD guy like me can write a book.

few times before switching to a regular bat and coming up to the plate. When the player swings the light bat, they're still set up to swing the heavy one, and the result is that the ball flies much farther. The same is true of speed. Try driving fast on the highway; then, pull off on a slow street and feel the difference. It seems like you are crawling. We can use this to hack the brain into reading faster simply by overclocking our regular reading ability.

To Speed-Read, Follow These Steps

Step One: Get comfortable reading with your finger as a guide.

Step Two: Simulate the process of reading in short intervals of two to three minutes. Take breaks in between.

Step Three: Test your reading speed again.

Note: there are programs that claim to teach subconscious or instant image-based reading ability. I have seen no credible proof that they work. Use objective data to confirm results, and with any program like this, if at any time you feel stress or strain in your eyes, stop and rest them. Don't overexert yourself, and always contact a medical professional if there is excessive or long-lasting discomfort.

For a full course on speed-reading, look at www.brainhackers.com. Use this book's proof of purchase for a discount.

CHAPTER **SUMMARY**

- Knowing that our brain uses comparison to measure things like speed, we can trick it to read faster by changing our objects of comparison.
- Practicing the three steps in this Axiom will get you speed-reading more quickly than you ever thought!

AXIOM SIX

ENCODING

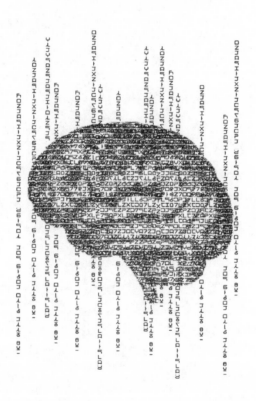

Our brains can only store and process information in terms of our senses. For example, we can memorize a list of objects by visualizing them around the room, but can't do that with numbers. By using a code, we can turn these numbers into other objects, making them easy to link.

The art of code making is a big part of brainhacking.

14 | A Head for Numbers

In my fourth year of high school, I came home to find my family gathered around the TV. My mom, dad, and sister were all staring at it with fascination.

"Take a look, David," my mother said with a smile, waving me over. "Look what your father did."

Sitting on top of the TV was a tiny metal tin held down by duct tape. The box said "Sucrets," a popular breath mint that came in a metal tin. Coming from the box was a series of tentacle-like wires tracing back behind the TV. My dad stood triumphantly beside the TV with his hand poised over the tiny box with his finger on the switch at the side.

On the screen, the TV showed one of the many pay-per-view channels cable had to offer at the time. This was new technology. Basically, the cable company would scramble the signal of all these channels to non-customers to make it almost impossible to make out what was happening on the screen.

There were movie channels, sports, and of course the adult channels. Every kid my age was curious to switch to the adult channel, hoping to see something exciting, but it was impossible to tell what was happening on the screen. The picture was so scrambled, a human body would be almost unrecognizable. It was like an extreme electronic Picasso mixing up and twisting everything. For example, the channel he was showing me was clearly a Disney movie, but I could only vaguely make out the color and shape of the images.

"Okay, Dave. Look at the screen," he said, gesturing to the scrambled scene as he flipped the switch.

Suddenly, the scene unscrambled, and we could see the movie in crystal clarity. It was incredible.

"How did you do that?" I asked

"Oh, I saw a schematic in *Popular Electronics* and got the parts at Radio Shack. There's nothing you can't do if you put your mind to it," he replied.

"Aren't we breaking the law?" my sister, Kathy, asked.

"Well, the cable company is sending me that signal. What I do with it is up to me, I think. Besides, sometimes rules are meant to be broken, especially when the cable company is charging eight bucks a movie."

My mother gave me a worried look, afraid they were teaching a bad lesson to the kids. But I just smiled. This felt like an answer to my problem.

MEMORY CODES

There are two different kinds of information when it comes to memory brainhacks. The first type is physical/visual information—like a list of groceries or objects. We can easily recall this by making a mental journey (Journey Brainhack on page 24) out of them.

The second is abstract information. This includes anything we can't visualize and thus does not easily fit into our mental journey. These are things like numbers, formulas, addresses, technical terms, languages, playing cards, and more. We will cover how to memorize complex words and terms in a later section on languages and sub-words. The rest of the abstract information can be memorized using memory codes.

Visual Codes

The simplest and most direct memory code is the visual code. Take any information you need to memorize, and if it can be turned into a picture directly based on how it looks, it can be a visual code.

Ancients did this to the night sky to remember the positions of the stars. It would be impossible to commit to memory every star, but make them into animals and gods performing a scene, and it sticks in the mind. Astrology is a mnemonic device.

. The most common visual code today is for numbers. Let's say I wanted to memorize a list of ten things, but I wanted to recall their position without having to count from the beginning. Think of top ten lists, for example. Make a visual image out of each number. 1 becomes a stick, 2 becomes a swan (do you see it?), 3 is a comb or pitchfork, 4 is a flamingo with one leg up. And so on. Then link each item in the top ten list to the right object and you will recall the position perfectly every time. This can be a simple way to memorize numbers.

Alphabet Code

Sometimes a code is a simple rule, like the code to memorize letters in the alphabet (like in a license plate or when memorizing a Canadian postal code). Simply pick the smallest word you can that starts with or sounds like the letter.

For me, the letter A is The Fonz, from *Happy Days*, saying his catch-phrase (having to explain this makes me feel old); B is a bee; C is the sea; and so on. Pick your own words. The simpler the better.

The other rule of code making is to use the same code every time. Don't use a BB gun for the letter B if you've already decided to use the insect. It will get very confusing very fast.

This is just the tip of the iceberg though. There are codes I use to memorize multiple sets of numbers and cards all in one link. But start with the basics.

Here is how I came up with the simplest code for numbers in use today.

THE NUMERIC SPECTRUM©

I stared at some of the components in my dad's electronics box beside the TV. Then, it hit me. There was a special color code for resistors and other tiny components. When repairing electric circuits, they needed a way to label components so they could be read from a distance and any angle. So, they turned the numbers into colors and made little bands around each component. Now you could open a case and with just a tiny glance at a resistor, you could tell its value without removing it to read a serial number.

Memorize Numbers the Easy Way

When I was seventeen, I created the numeric spectrum technique as a simple way to memorize numbers.

Inspired by electronic resistor codes, it's highly intuitive and only takes minutes to learn.

The numbers from 9 to 0 are given colors in the order of the rainbow:

0 = Black or White

1 = Red

2 = Orange

3 = Yellow

4 = Green

5 = Blue

6 = Purple

7 = Brown (the dirt at the end of the rainbow)

8 = Silver (the pot at the end of the rainbow)

9 = Gold (the treasure inside it)

After learning the code, you need a simple way to connect the numbers to the corresponding colors in your mind. Instead of memorizing them by linking separate items together, these colors can just be added in order to a mental movie. Using a color code gives us so many choices when memorizing that we don't need a journey or a series of links—just one continuous movie in your mind. I call this type of memorization stringing, because it's smoother than making links in a chain.

Let's use our newfound brainhack to memorize pi.

Here is the number: 3.1415926535 . . .

I like to start with a link to what we are memorizing, so I will think of a pie—a *yellow* pie for the number three. Then, to string memories, just play a game of add-on, adding the next number (color) to the last one. Just pick an object that is that color. Here is what I thought of.

3 A yellow pie

1 A red fire hydrant the pie is sitting on

4 Green grass around the hydrant

1 Red roses growing from the green grass

5 Blue water being sprayed on the roses

9 To add the new item my eye follows the water stream up to a golden nozzle on the end of the hose.

2 An orange garden hose attached to the nozzle

6 At this point, I got creative and imagined a purple monster holding the hose

5 A blue jay on the monster's shoulder

3 The yellow sun the jay flies into

8 Silver rain clouds that touch the sun

and keep going . . .

This can be done with any length of number, even thousands of digits, and it's just the tip of the iceberg.

> I used this technique to memorize one hundred digits of PI and earn extra credit from my math teacher—and I even convinced a new person to join the memory club at the same time! I have used and created many more codes over the years to learn everything from binary to Morse code, programming to formulas, and, of course, playing cards (covered in the next chapter).

I could make a color code for numbers and simplify the process. Instead of linking items together or using a journey that people had to learn in advance, I could paint a picture with the numbers using a few simple rules.

By the next memory club meeting, I had my new code—the numeric spectrum—and a new technique: stringing (as opposed to linking). It was much easier to teach, and people were able to use it to start memorizing hundreds of numbers after just a few minutes of training, making it still, to this day, the quickest number-learning technique.

At one time, I saw my education as someone else's responsibility. The system was meant to teach me, and it was not suited to the job. Only, the reality of education for me felt like I was watching a twisted movie. At this point, I decided it was *my* job to untwist it. I would be resourceful because some day I would not have educators around to show me things. I had to become my own teacher.

If you struggle with learning or memory, realize that for some of us, information is sometimes like a scrambled cable television channel. It's all about encoding, decoding, and connecting.

You're not broken. Things just need to be unscrambled.

CHAPTER **SUMMARY**

- Codes are used on information that is hard to visualize. The simplest version of this is to simply make objects out of abstract items based on how they look. Make a list of the information you want to turn into a code, and then use your imagination to think of images that fit. Have fun with it.

- A simple code for numbers is the visual code. Take each number and think of something it looks like. For example: 1 = stick, 2 = swan, 3 = pitchfork, 4 = sailboat, 5 = unicycle.

- To memorize letters, a simple code is to pick the most obvious word that starts with that letter: A = apple, B = bee.

- My color code for numbers is simple: 1 = red, 2 = orange, 3 = yellow, 4 = green, 5 = blue, 6 = purple, 7 = brown, 8 = silver, 9 = gold, 0 = black or white

- With my color code, there is no need to make a separate link or location for each number. Just string together items in a scene that makes sense.

15 | Memorize Playing Cards

In my last year of high school, a friend showed me an old copy of *The Guinness Book of Records* where a guy named Dominic O'Brien memorized six decks of cards on a Japanese TV show to set a record in 1985 (a record that has been broken many times since). I thought I could break that record with the right code for card memory. But I thought I would start smaller. So I did a charity event.

I got permission to make the event into an official charity drive at my high school that would raise money for the local United Way. My friends and I asked people to pledge to pay an amount per card that I recalled. Some pledged a dime or quarter, but a few pledged five dollars or more, thinking I would only recall ten or fifteen cards. This was going to be a surprise for them.

To prepare for the event, I turned to my friend Scott for advice. At this point, Scott was already a professional magician, from a long line of magicians. He was performing on stage with his dad before he could walk. So, he knew a few things about cards and performances. In fact, many of today's memory codes originated on stages with magicians.

(It was cool having a magician friend, because it's the only other job that is as weird as memory expert. I remember one time in my twenties, Scott and I were going to a night club with my martial arts instructor and good friend Asaad. I stopped them and said, "Wait, guys, we need a cover story. No one is going to believe a magician, a memory expert, and a kung fu master walked into a bar. It sounds like the setup for a joke.")

Scott was the perfect person to help me prepare. His advice was to aim higher than the task called for and to practice offstage before the event.

"When you're onstage, everything will happen so fast, and if you're not careful, nerves will stress you out and make you make mistakes," he said. "So, the top magicians in the world practice a trick to the point of being able to do it in their sleep. Literally. One of the cues that you're ready to perform comes when you dream about doing the magic trick from beginning to end."

It was good advice to overprepare. However, there are some things you never learn until they happen.

The next piece of advice was to get a good strategy. "Every magician learns the basic tricks," he said, "but they start to create their own style, tricks, and props. Like you did when you invented new memory techniques. That's like when a magician gets good enough to reinvent the art and fool other magicians."

If I was going to do well at memorizing cards, I knew I needed to make my own code.

THE VISUAL CARD CODE

To memorize something that you can't visualize, you often need a code to translate the information into something you can imagine. This concept is similar to how computers turn images into thousands of numbers in order to store them. To us, numbers are tough to remember, but to a computer, images are difficult, so the code is used to translate back and forth. The better the code, the easier it is to store and use the information.

At the time, existing codes for memorizing cards were complex, requiring hours, even weeks, of study and training to memorize a full deck of cards quickly.

On the day of the charity event, my friends Jo and Scott were there to motivate me, and so was the news station CKCO in Kitchener, Ontario.

The Quickest Card Code to Learn

My code needed to have as simple a process as possible to translate the cards into an image I can link in a journey. So, I started looking at the cards. I flipped card after card, looking for inspiration, and then stopped on one card. The eight of hearts: I saw something in it. It was just a glimpse of pattern recognition, like when you see a cloud that looks like a bird or a face in a piece of burnt toast. I looked at the eight of hearts and saw an ice cream cone.

The answer was to make a visual card code! So far, this had only been done for numbers. Like how a 2 looked like a swan, and a 3 could be a pitchfork. No one had tried it for cards. I grabbed my pen and went to work. With this new code in my mind, I flipped through the cards, and in a few minutes, I had mastered the code and could memorize a deck with it.

Previously, it took me weeks to make my code second nature, only to forget it. But with this code, even when I stopped practicing, it took only minutes to learn and master this visual card code again. Now, it's almost impossible to forget, because every card object looks like the card's top corner.

Try it yourself. Take a look at the following card images and make a funny or unique mental journey with them.

The complete card code list is found at www.brainhackers.com.

It was late in the day, after everyone had gone home, and the school was almost empty aside from us. We were in the cafeteria, with the six decks of cards laid out in front of me. A rush of excitement filled me, but the nerves were present too. I blinked a few times and breathed out to focus. Jo and Scott sat close, nodding with encouragement.

I quickly got to work, flipping card after card and linking the image to a location in my mind.

I went through the first three decks and had to take a break to talk to the media a bit. Then, I finished up the memorization and started to recall.

Multiple witnesses watched me recite the cards one at a time, and it was at that point that the laughs turned to stunned faces. I didn't recall just ten or twenty cards, but hundreds. Out of 312 cards, I identified almost three hundred correctly. Not good enough for a Guinness Record, but very good.

Earlier that day, I had discovered that the current Guinness Record for this event had jumped to forty decks of cards, not even close to six anymore. And, I reasoned, if I were to attempt the world record, I would have needed to be registered in advance anyways. Record hopes aside, this charity event changed my life more than anything up until that point. I include it in this book so it might inspire some readers to try something big. For everyone who shot for the moon or climbed the tallest mountain, there was a moment like this that was a turning point. It was the first time I really pushed my limits, and others saw the result, shedding the doubt I'd always let plague the back of my mind. I learned that day that a big demonstration changes everything about how people look at you.

The teachers who saw the event changed their tune, and aside from Mr. Ross, they never called me a cheater again—or made me redo tests. My grades were adjusted to reflect the actual test scores I had earned.

The news media were also amazed. So much so that they wanted to return the next day with a camera crew to test me again. This event gave me confidence in the knowledge that I could change my brain and how others saw me. I had to go further than anyone else expected, but aiming high paid off.

As a bonus, it was also nice to raise money for charity. I had more than a few interesting conversations with donors who had promised a high dollar amount per card, assuming they wouldn't pay much. To say they were displeased to find out they owed hundreds of times more money than they'd imagined would be an understatement. We weren't heartless, though. We reduced each amount to a reasonable sum so people could still feel good about paying. Altogether, we raised over four thousand dollars, and some respect to boot. It was a good start.

CHAPTER **SUMMARY**

- The fastest card code to learn is this visual code. With a little practice it can be mastered in as little as one night. Each card is a number and suit, so I made a mental image of how it looked in the top left corner.

INTELLIGENCE HAS MULTIPLE SIDES AND CAN BE CHANGED

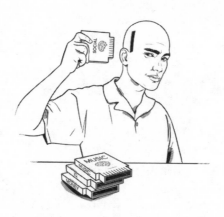

A book on brainhacks would be incomplete without the biggest brainhack of them all: hacks to become smarter. There is a common belief that IQ is born and cannot be changed, but brainhackers around the world are proving them wrong. Not only can you improve IQ with strategy and training, but there are also many other brainhacks that unleash great ability to solve problems and understand concepts better.

Also, mastering skills like deductive and inductive reasoning, multiple intelligences, EQ, game theory, logic, and more will give you an advantage in nearly every area of life.

16 | Which Intelligence Do I Hack?

It was parent-teacher night in my second year of high school. I had already made a lot of improvement in my grades, and my debate club had recently shifted into a memory club, so even though I hadn't achieved success as great as my card memorization trick yet, my memory techniques were just starting to become well-known. Overall, school was going well, and I was running ahead to the gym with my parents trailing behind, looking forward to hearing what my teachers had to say. I turned a corner at full speed and bumped right into the looming Mr. Ross.

"David, you are unfocused and out of control. Don't run in the hallways, and bring me to your parents. If I can't talk sense into you, I can at least talk sense into them," he said as my mom turned around the corner, hearing every word.

He gestured for them to come to his table and sit down to "talk sense" into my parents.

"Mr. and Mrs. Farrow, we all know what David did with his tests was impossible. Your son is cheating. In all my years teaching, I have never once seen such a spike in grades from an honest student. A transformation like that, from a poor learner to a great learner, is simply not possible."

"Not with that attitude," my mom replied.

Mr. Ross continued with his defeatist platitudes. "Growing up is about accepting the cards that we're dealt and learning to live with them," he explained. "The brain is hardwired by this age, and it doesn't change. As educators, it's our job to prepare students for the life they are best suited for. Your son could be a good tradesman."

My mother held her temper but responded coolly. "My son has chronic pain in his back. He can't be working in a physically demanding job as he gets older. My husband works in a factory; I know what that does to your body."

My dad added, "It sounds like you've given up on these kids before giving them a chance to figure things out."

"The sooner David accepts that he has disabilities that cannot be overcome, the sooner he can put his life on track," Ross replied.

"On track to the poor house, you mean," my mother retorted. I was proud of her at that moment. She continued, "What's the point of education if effort doesn't make a difference? If success is only luck, then why even *have* teachers?"

Frustrated, Mr. Ross tried to prove his point by talking to me. "David, you get distracted easily, right?"

"Sometimes, but other times I am so focused on a video game or TV show, no one can pull me away."

Mr. Ross grunted. "Well, that's called hyperfocus, and it only happens in ADHD kids for things that are entertaining, like TV. That won't help you in school."

I said, "What if I make school more entertaining? What if I make a game out of it?"

"Education isn't a game. That's one of the most ridiculous things I've ever heard," he said.

"Did you ever think that the system could be wrong? History is written by the winners, not the losers, and the curriculum you follow, and all your education theories are written by the winners of this system. The winners think the education system works because it worked for them. But if you learn a different way or you just lack study skills, you're a failure instead of different. I don't think dyslexia and ADHD always have to be disadvantages."

Ross missed the point and couldn't imagine these so-called disadvantages could actually have advantages; he took my attempt to challenge the system as a challenge to the diagnosis.

"Well," said Mr. Ross, "that's wrong. You were diagnosed correctly."

I realized we were having two different conversations. So I tried to explain again.

"I'm aware I think differently than others, but I'm saying that dyslexia and ADHD are not really disabilities because reading and studying aren't natural abilities to begin with. They're skills that are learned. With practice and solid strategies, we can become smarter, improve our memory, and train our brain to do almost anything, with or without dyslexia and ADHD," I said. My parents smiled supportively.

"That's not true," Mr. Ross snapped. "Some are better at studying than others. There is a natural talent, and you can't change that. Your ADHD means you can't focus without medication, and your dyslexia means you lack the ability to read properly—that is simply what it means."

"But reading isn't a natural ability. It's a skill. Ditto learning—and test-taking," I replied.

I tried to get my point across another way. I explained that if you gave babies all the books in the world, they would never learn to read without instruction. But they do learn to walk on their own. Saying I have a learning or reading disability is like saying a person has a basketball disability because they can't dribble or do a layup. Maybe you should tell kids to play the game differently. Maybe I can't jump, but I can shoot three-pointers.

He stared at me with his mouth open in disbelief.

So, I tried to explain my analogy. "Like instead of basketball, it's reading, and maybe I approach the problem differently, and—"

At this point, Mr. Ross lost any façade of calm. "Yes, I understood your analogy. What I'm amazed by is the denial and delusion here. You have ADHD and dyslexia. You will never be a genius, and you'll never run your own company like you want to. I keep trying to tell you: If you ever want to be successful, and if you ever want to achieve your goals, you need to aim lower." He turned to my mother.

"Mrs. Farrow, you need to stop encouraging this kind of thing. He thinks he knows better than professionals with degrees and years of training. I've been a certified Ontario teacher for years. I take every training opportunity to improve my skills, year in and year out, and your son constantly undermines me by trying to *lecture* me about education," Mr. Ross said.

My dad stepped in. "Be honest. You take that extra training because your union deal raises your pay each time. It's not for the kids."

My dad was what they called street-smart. He didn't like to have academics talking down to him, especially when he was the person most people would call when anything broke. Just because my dad had different skills than an academic, that didn't mean that he wasn't smart. Momentarily distracted, I became absorbed in thinking about what it means to be smart.

TESTING THE BRAIN

Since the dawn of time, humans have tried to figure out which of us is the cleverest. Yet, many brain tests have been little better than an astrology chart when it comes to predicting performance.

IQ tests have a troubled history as well, and though they are based on science, they're far from the only indicator of success in life. For example, one of the highest IQs ever recorded belonged to a man named Christopher Langan, who worked for much of his life as a bouncer.

Tests like the Big Five (or OCEAN) personality test are fantastic for discovering your personality and thus what you want to do, but how do we know what we're good at? Today, the theory of multiple intelligences seems to be the most useful in helping people prosper. As it turns out, the idea that we all have strengths and weaknesses is confirmed by science. If the goal of education is to prepare us for the future, then multiple intelligences is the measuring stick we ought to use en route.

MULTIPLE INTELLIGENCES

How smart are you? There are multiple kinds of intelligence:

1. **Pure IQ**—Ability to solve problems, usually of a logical nature (also known as logical intelligence)
2. **Spatial**—Ability to visualize the 3D world
3. **Musical**—Ability to discern sounds or pitch
4. **Interpersonal**—Ability to communicate with and motivate people
5. **Bodily**—Ability to coordinate between the body and brain
6. **Linguistic**—Ability to articulate thoughts and ideas well
7. **Intrapersonal**—Ability to achieve self-awareness
8. **Naturalist**—Ability to understand living things and growth
9. **Existential**—Ability to understand philosophical questions
10. **Emotional intelligence**—Ability to self-regulate; demonstrates social skills and empathy
11. **Financial intelligence**—Ability to understand how humans and things of value interact

All of these abilities can be improved with practice. However, the most important type of intelligence to me is wisdom. This is my definition of wisdom:

12. **Wisdom**—The ability to learn from the past to guide the future. I believe all intelligences should lead to wisdom.

The conversation was winding down, and as it went on, my parents seemed less argumentative and more open to Mr. Ross's words. My mother concluded the meeting by thanking him for his opinion and his time.

I felt a cloud of doubt filling me as I walked away from the table—like I had won a battle in my mind but had bitten the hand that could feed me grades and change my direction. Maybe everything he said was true, and I knew nothing about the brain. Maybe I was just delusional. I passed a poster for *Man of La Mancha*, a school play coming up. I had a small speaking part in it, and in that moment, wondered if I was like

Don Quixote. *I think I'm a knight on the holy quest . . . but maybe I'm just chasing windmills?*

We all stopped to bundle up with hats, gloves, and coats to face the Canadian cold.

"I'll warm up the car," my dad said as he walked ahead.

My mom stood there. She never went to college and was raised in an orphanage, so she knew what it was like to get a rocky start in life. In fact, she had some pretty crazy ideas about religion that I didn't agree with at the time, but when she turned to me, her words seemed to come from another place. A part deep inside that she was tapping into. "You don't believe a damn word that man says." (Only, she didn't say *damn*; she said something worse . . . or better.)

She paused.

"You're smart, but your brain thinks differently. You keep searching for a way to learn that works for you," she said, her expression fierce.

That was all I needed. Throughout the next few years of high school, when someone like Mr. Ross told me I would never succeed, or I wouldn't amount to anything, all I had to do was think about my mother's face in that moment.

Intelligence Hierarchy Hack

If we want to raise our intelligence, we need to be better at solving problems. The biggest mistake people make when trying to solve a problem—from an escape room to a debate—is to not use their best skills. For most problems, there are multiple ways to find the solution, but we get stuck in the way we think they should be solved. To fix this, make an intelligence hierarchy.

Write down the types of intelligences above in order of what you are best at. This will create your own personal list of skills, and the next time you encounter a problem, you will be able to turn to your strongest tools first.

CHAPTER **SUMMARY**

- There are more ways to measure intelligence than just IQ. The world is complex, so everyone has strengths and weaknesses. What are you good at?
- With the Intelligence Hierarchy Hack, look at the list of intelligences and put them in order of what is your strongest to weakest. This will give you the ability to find your best path in life.

17 | Learning Strategies, Not Styles

After the charity event, I was given a new device to fidget with. A label maker. I was pretty messy (a common trait of ADHD), so the label maker was to encourage me to get organized. Of course, I fiddled around with it in class.

It was a small plastic device that looked like a cheap phaser, with a dial on top and a trigger on the bottom. I would turn the dial on top of a letter I wanted to label and then pull the trigger. It would emboss that letter into a strip of black plastic inside, turning the letter white and moving the strip forward a bit. By repeating the process, I could make a sticker label for any word I wanted.

I was sitting in Mr. Ross's class, trying to make some labels, when the announcement sounded.

"Dave Farrow to the office, please," the speakers bellowed.

Mr. Ross's gaze turned to me. "You're in trouble now, David," he said, then noticed the labels I was applying to the desk. "And what do you think you're doing damaging school property?"

Another student said, "I don't think he's in trouble. It's about the cards he memorized for charity."

"Don't be ridiculous," Ross replied. "This memory stuff is obviously a trick. They only work for him because he is a visual learner."

I'd had enough. "A few weeks ago, you called these memory techniques cheating," I replied. "And you said I was a kinesthetic learner. That's another one of those educational theories without data to back it up."

* * *

The notion of learning styles is another great example of the many groundless "learning theories" pushed in classrooms worldwide. It's the result of a system that often mistakes experienced opinions for actual data.

Created by Neil Fleming, a wildly famous professor, the theory of learning styles is called VARK (Visual; Aural, or auditory; Reading and writing; Kinesthetic). It's an attempt to sort kids based on the way they learn, and it makes some intuitive sense. Some of us tend to like lectures (auditory), and others don't understand things until they see a diagram (visual). Others like to take action and touch the lessons (kinesthetic). Fleming's theory rapidly spread through education systems worldwide because it seemed to give teachers what they wanted—a kid-sized sorting hat.

When this system combined with natural biases, students scoring high in kinesthetic learning were encouraged away from intellectual subjects and pushed into trades. Thus, it seemed that education finally had a scientific way to separate all the intellectuals from the working class in society.

The only problem is, it's false. Time and time again, researchers have tried to prove this theory, and it doesn't hold up. The same child that scores high in kinesthetic learning one day will score higher in visual learning another day. The core of this theory and other "educational sorting hat" ideas is to take learning strategies we use and create identities out of them—mistaking a tool we use for a thing we are. The result of attempts like this can disenfranchise the learner. Meanwhile, we can take this attempt at label making and turn it into an empowering strategy.

SPEED COMPREHENSION WITH LEARNING STRATEGIES

When I first learned how to drive, I wanted to start with a manual transmission. It was going badly. The instructor told me the instructions one step at a time.

"Flip this switch . . . turn the knob . . . press the clutch . . . get in gear . . . check the mirror . . . and release the clutch . . ." And apparently the last step was to grind the gears, making the car scream in pain, because that's what happened.

Despite my protests, the instructor just kept ticking off commands with no awareness of my difficulties. To her credit, many people said they learned perfectly well with her help and this step-by-step process was just fine for them. Not me.

I called my dad for help and in ten minutes, he described how a manual transmission clutch worked, and as I visualized it, everything became clear. He said a clutch is basically two plates of metal—one connected to the wheels and one to the engine. When I press the clutch, I separate the pieces making it possible to change gears, and then letting go of the clutch brings the plates together, moving the car forward.

It only took few minutes of getting a feel for the clutch, and I was driving smoothly. So, I'm a visual learner, right? But wait—the information was told to me on the phone, so am I auditory? Neither. These are no more than mislabeled versions of real learning strategies we all use.

The three categories of learning are probably better described as follows:

1. global (big picture)
2. linear (sequential or step-by-step instructions)
3. kinesthetic (trial and error)

The so-called visual learner is actually trying to see the big picture first before diving into the details. They want to see how something works before exploring the minutiae involved.

The so-called auditory learner is actually using a sequential strategy, learning the step-by-step process to acquire an understanding of a subject.

Meanwhile, the kinesthetic learner is about trial and error. This may seem ineffective until you realize that most inventions and tech startups use this approach.

The secret is: These are tools we all use. Everyone uses trial and error, big-picture thinking, and step-by-step instruction in different situations. In this case, step-by-step thinking didn't work for me because I'm curious about how mechanical things work. Someone else without that curiosity would probably be okay learning a step-by-step approach. We can have a preference, but the problem comes when we take a natural learning tool and attach an identity to it.

If you think of yourself as a trial-and-error learner, then try to assemble an Ikea bookshelf. You'll soon become a sequential thinker, in the same way that I'm left-handed but use a mouse with my right hand because every computer in the world puts the mouse on the right side. Just being aware of these strategies will make you smarter and better able to solve problems. The next time you're stuck, switch strategies.

A LABEL THAT STICKS

Back in the class, I waited impatiently for Mr. Ross to finish so I could head to the office. But Mr. Ross continued. "Kinesthetic learners work with their hands; they're the basic labor force in this world. They can specialize in things like plumbing or carpentry. This is just how the system works; there's no use trying to get around it. You can't cheat the system."

I turned the dial a few times and spelled the word *cheat*, then stuck it to the desk.

"The visual people are creative, and that doesn't often pay the bills. Hence, they need to learn to adapt or fail. Like if they have ADHD, they need to be realistic."

I punched out the letters *ADHD* and stuck the label on the desk.

"The auditory learners can succeed in lectures; they enter higher education and become the intellectuals."

"It's interesting," I replied. "It's interesting that you are at the top of that unbiased imaginary intellectual system, right?"

I was punching out another label when he jumped in.

"Stop right there, Mr. Farrow. Before you go to the office, explain what you are doing damaging that desk?"

For years, I had been hounded by this man. Every time he attacked, I would get upset or emotional. Instead, I decided to reframe the situation.

Reframing Hack

We compare all our experiences to things around us. How much money we make, or how well we dress, or how funny we think we are at parties—these are all judged in comparison to those around us. In the quest to get smarter, it's helpful to change this frame of reference sometimes. It can make you see a solution to your problems as well as win a debate.

With Mr. Ross, I decided to reframe his argument using my new fidget device.

"I was given this gift, and it made me think about logical fallacies." I held up the label maker. "Those dirty tricks people like to use in arguments to avoid addressing the facts the other person is presenting."

I explained the "straw man" argument, where you misrepresent your opponent's ideas to make them an easier target, and "ad hominem," where you attack the person instead of their ideas.

"What's your point?" he responded.

"You are using a logical fallacy I call *label making*," I said with a smile, holding up the little device in my hand. "Instead of criticizing my brainhacks and the studying strategies I'm developing, you try to distract from their success by placing labels on me. Some are real, like 'ADHD,' but most of your labels just don't stick . . . like how these labels just peel right off the desk."

Don't Let Labels Stick Hack

Today, politics across the board have generally devolved into label making. When a label maker tries to win an argument by throwing labels at you or others, don't let them stick. Reframe the label maker's point by asking why they need to label rather than engage. Ask what proof they have. If we all invite debate rather than settling for divisive labels, it may start to reverse the huge divide in today's society.

Mr. Ross's mouth twitched in response. So, I decided to reframe the argument before he could strike. "So, that's why you are a label maker— you want to reinforce your beliefs through labels. You want to reinforce your own labels—your credentials. Instead of just being a good teacher and letting the results speak for themselves, you need to reinforce those labels to make sure you are above me as an educator."

"I *am* above you as an educator," he said.

"Then do something better than criticizing students for working to improve their grades." I stood up, planning to leave for the principal's office.

There was a knock at the door. Outside was a cameraman and reporter from the local TV station, who must have gotten tired of waiting at the office.

They leaned into the class. "We want to talk to the memory whiz kid," they said.

Mr. Ross's jaw dropped.

I said to Mr. Ross, "I'm going to go out and get a label that will stick, and I don't care how tough it is. If another person can do a thing, I can figure out how to do it too."

As I stood up and walked to the reporter, Mr. Ross went to my desk, peeling off the labels he had tried to apply to me.

Trick, ADHD, cheat. Then one label gave him trouble. It just would not come off no matter how much he pried it with his nail.

Guinness.

CHAPTER **SUMMARY**

- The popular concept of learning styles is flawed, restricting people to one method and one sense. In reality, we all use each of these strategies and styles in different situations. Instead, these are the three main learning strategies people fall back on:
  1. **Global (big picture):** Getting a clear picture of the entire process. Look at it from twenty thousand feet. Then, zoom in to learn the details. Limitation: You can miss details and think you know more than you do.
  2. **Linear (sequential or step-by-step instructions):** The fastest way between two points is a straight line, and duplicating others' instructions is the fastest way to perform an established task. Limitation: This is not helpful with new discoveries or subjects with multiple results.
  3. **Kinesthetic (trial and error):** Jumping in to work on a project without learning the basics or hearing instructions is unwise for a math test. But learning by doing so has yielded nearly every major discovery in science and engineering. Limitation: You can waste a lot of time doing the wrong thing. New start-ups call this process, "fail fast, and fail often."
- Today it seems that everyone uses logical fallacies to try and mic drop their political opponents. Bring back civil debates by reframing the debate. People prefer a rational debate to spiteful name calling. The label maker tries to avoid a debate by blanketing their opponent with a label. Peel it off and reframe the conversation.

AXIOM EIGHT
THE SKILL OF FOCUS

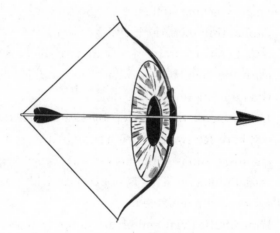

As I've said previously, the brain is the most powerful computer with the least powerful battery. What we call focus, flow, or being in the zone is all a tool of evolution to give us an advantage when the stakes are high.

Focus occurs on a spectrum between bored and stressed, and we can never know for sure if we have achieved it until after it's over. When you understand that you are trying to study for a test using a mechanism built to hunt an elephant, everything makes more sense.

Here, we will learn how to control our peak focus state by understanding the first thought mechanism, the questioning mind, and the deadline reaction. With these skills combined, it is possible to achieve superhuman focus for hours without fatigue.

18 | It's Fight or Flight

A young woman came up to me in tears after a summer memory camp I taught in Florida recently. She reminded me of myself at fourteen. She told me that she took a medication for ADHD that removed her appetite, so five days a week, she took it and starved. Then, her mother helped to force-feed her on weekends to get enough calories to combat her lack of appetite during the week. Hearing about the entire process left me speechless and horrified.

My heart was on the floor but bounced back up when she told me how the focus technique covered in this section changed everything. Now she could focus using a strategy and not just drugs—this gave her hope and changed her life.

Another time, someone came up to me after I spoke at a college in Georgia, telling me privately that they had been failing and not planning to return the following year. Then, they said, my focus technique changed everything. Instead of quitting, they turned their grades around and graduated.

If you follow along with the instructions and master the hacks in this chapter, you will control the most elusive and sought-after state of mind: focus.

It happens to all of us. We think we're paying attention to a lecture or what we're reading, only to suddenly realize we've been staring at the same spot for five minutes, zoning out. In my early years of high school, I tried everything, but none of it was successful in raising my grades. I tried drinking lots of coffee and energy drinks to stay alert, hoping for focus, but nothing helped.

COGNITIVE SELF-DECEPTION

So, I went back to first principles. This is a way of thinking that was recently popularized by Elon Musk. The idea is that in most situations when you want to solve a problem, the best strategy is to find another person who has done it already and emulate them. But when there is no model and you're experiencing something new, it's best to go back to basics and start with what you know.

This was in the early days of ADHD diagnosis. At the time, there were several scandals publicized about experts overdiagnosing or misdiagnosing kids, often in response to incentives by the education system. In addition to diagnosis, there was a lot of debate as to the proper strategy to teach those with ADHD.

I knew that I needed to take the reins on my own education, and to do that, I needed data. I tried to count the number of times I got distracted while trying to study—even if it was only for a few seconds. When I lost focus, I marked it down and took a break. But then, a new problem came up. The brain is self-deceptive when it comes to cognitive functions. That means that when our own brain is failing at a task, it often takes steps to convince us that everything is okay. We see this with Alzheimer's patients. The vast majority of patients are brought to doctors by loved ones, and think they don't have a problem despite having many symptoms. The brain convinces us that these are normal or completely blocks it out. Think of a time you tried to argue with someone who was struggling with depression or addiction. It can feel like the solution is right in front of you, clear as day, but they can't see it. One of the reasons for this is that the brain itself can block difficult realities from our awareness.

Same too with focus and productivity. We are terrible at being able to tell if we are actually focusing or getting distracted, or how productive we're actually being. I noticed this when I started practicing card memorization for my charity event.

I realized that I always started making mistakes recalling cards at the same time: right at the ten-minute mark! Nearly every time I tried to memorize cards for more than ten minutes in a row, I would make a mistake on a few cards; then, more mistakes would follow. I tested this on classmates in my memory club and found they did the same thing. So, this time limit on focus was consistent. But why?

THE MEMORY CURVE

In high school, researching studies on focus, I came across the idea of the memory curve. It's a memory concept more researched than nearly any other cognitive principle I could find. It's a chart showing the average amount of material people can recall at different points in a study session. When charted out, it follows a curve where, as you would expect, people are fresh and score high at the beginning of a study session, then lose focus over time. Still, when the study session is about to end, the brain wakes up again, and the line goes back up, making a flat-bottomed U-shape.

Students were asked to memorize information over a long period of two to four hours, with new information being presented at periodic intervals. Then, they were asked to recall the information, and the scores followed a clear pattern. Everyone had a high recall for the thing they learned first. This is odd because that information was learned longest ago from the test! After ten minutes' worth of study material, people thought they continued to score well, but recall dropped quickly to 10% on average. It stayed there until the end of the session, where it jumps back up to 90% for the last ten minutes' study material.

This concept, also known as primacy and recency, is supported by a lot of data in many different studies. I believe universities should make all their studies and data available to the public, because thousands of people like me are trying to figure out problems like this. (However, I am also fairly cynical about academia, and especially its insular nature. I think this was why I chose to take an entrepreneurial approach to life rather than the academic route. I was trying to figure out my brain to improve my life, so my approach was practical.)

Seeing real data makes a difference. When I saw the data from actual studies, it became clear to me that the memory curve wasn't a curve at all but a cliff. By combining the data with what I had observed in my memory training, I realized that mainstream academia had reached the wrong conclusion about this data, and that conclusion had made all the difference in how science approached the art of memory.

The commonly accepted belief about this concept was that the brain places importance on the location of the information. Information we hear first and last is the most significant. There is also a belief that emotions help make memories stick more. These are interesting ideas, but not true in my experience.

What I saw was not a memory curve or primacy and recency. I saw the fight-or-flight response.

FOCUS IS JUST STRESS WITH A PURPOSE

We have been taught to think of stress as bad and the core of all ills in our society. This isn't too far from the truth. Stress influences and even causes most of what is thought of as modern ailments, from heart disease to cancer. But this is an oversimplification, because it's also responsible for every breakthrough and productive deadline reached. The only way to understand stress is to see it in the wild.

Imagine you're a hunter or gatherer living one hundred thousand years ago in a jungle. You spend most of your days doing leisurely activities, relaxing, grooming, and enjoying family. Then, one day, you see a tiger. Your brain immediately reacts, as does the tiger. The tiger will eat you, or you can jump in the river, and maybe the tiger gives up if you're lucky. Either way, this conflict, like all conflicts in the wild, will be over in minutes.

Nature is geared toward these short, powerful bursts of energy because that's the best solution for a conflict. No one is fighting the tiger an hour later. As a result of this evolutionary heritage, no animal can handle conflict or stress for an extended period, and neither can your brain.

PRIMARY AND RECENCY CHART

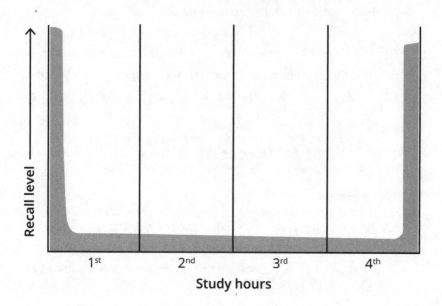

When I looked at the primacy and recency chart, I saw that the brain does very well at first, but shuts down to 10% of its normal activity within just five to ten minutes of memorizing something. That effect isn't about position or emotion. It comes from the quarter-of-a-billion-year-old history built into our genes—a system meant to handle specific challenges.

Yes, our brain is powerful and a force for civilization. It's the single most complex thing in the known universe, but, as I've said, it has a terrible battery. The minute we achieve a focused state, we have a brain chemistry–based timer counting down. You can count down the seconds until we run out of the stuff that makes us focus. This seems like a limitation, but in fact, it's beautiful. We've gone up against animals with claws, teeth, strength, and speed with nothing but our brains and the ability to focus. And we are still here. That's amazing!

DEADLINE PRINCIPLE BRAINHACK

The solution is to make it a game. I decided to create a series of timed intervals that were shorter than my ten-minute limits and set up the memory task to fit this timing rather than try to force my brain to focus for hours. The key to making this work is the deadline principle.

We get more focused as we get closer to a deadline. Think back to school when a teacher would give you a project that was due in six weeks. I'm betting you didn't go home that night to start working on it, but instead waited till the day before the deadline before your brain really got in gear.

The Focus-Burst™ Technique

Here are a few rules.

1. Break down your job, studies, or project into short chunks. Very short. Less than ten minutes each. This means one task at a time, like memorizing a few words or reviewing one page.

2. Set a goal for each short burst. Something you want to accomplish in this time.

3. Use an external timer that makes a noise at the end of the countdown. Don't just look up at the clock to see if your burst is done; you will never get fully immersed until you use a timer.

4. Make your focus time five to eight minutes at the most. Once you get to ten minutes, then the brain starts to lose focus. This may seem like very little time, but try it and see the magic.

5. Focus on the task with intensity. No distractions. Do only that task for that chunk of time, and try to do it with as much energy as you can.

6. The study burst should mimic a fight-or-flight situation. So, raise the intensity of the task by setting a big goal or something

that pushes you to work at your peak. Remember, for this to work we need to simulate danger or a fight in real life.

7. When the timer goes off, reset it for the same time (five to eight minutes), and relax for the same amount of time you did your burst. Just like the focus time seemed too short, this may seem like too much time, because we have been convinced that breaks should be short. This is not a factory, though—it's a machine in our heads that we want to keep running optimally. In my experience, this method gets three or more times the productivity of a short break and long focus, because it allows for your brain to fully reset and fully focus again. Do something fun or mentally low-intensity, like light reading or streaming a show. You're aiming for a full on and off switch.

8. Repeat the process.

Turns out there is a neurological phenomenon that happens when the deadline looms. The brain takes the task seriously. So, we just use a timer, and we replace the predators in the wild, but the brain still gets focused.

The result of these focus bursts was amazing. It worked. I was able to memorize for hours (in seven-minute intervals). I also discovered I would get twice the amount of work done in the same hour, even though half the time I was taking a break. That meant the focus burst was four times more productive than my usual pace.

As soon as I discovered this, I taught this to my classmates in the memory club, and their faces lit up. We used it for tasks like memorizing language class vocabulary, technical terms, and more, and every time they were amazed that they could memorize more information in one hour than they usually could in an entire day.

I did the same memory curve test that I'd seen in textbooks, but the results were different.

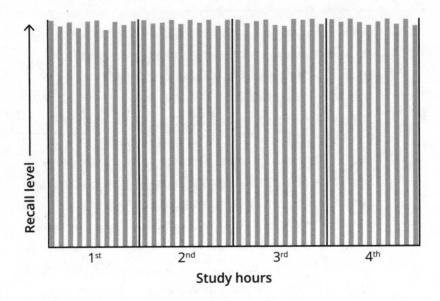

The gray parts represent my score on tests on the study material from each focus burst. It was clear that I could keep doing these focus bursts for hours without losing any focus. Now things were getting superhuman.

* * *

For those who want a technical explanation: When we do a focus burst, the amygdala tells the hypothalamus to trigger epinephrine (adrenaline) release into the body. This hormone raises heart rate and blood pressure slightly and opens airways, flooding the brain with oxygen. This makes you more alert, while your sight, hearing, and other senses become sharper, and your eyes focus and dilate faster. All of this happens in seconds, and you have this power for only precious minutes, so the brain is very selective about what causes it to activate. So, we need to make the focus burst intense. Then, during the break, your chemistry rebalances, letting you go back to 90% focus for another burst of energy later. Many think of focus like a laser. If that's true, it's more like a pulse laser or maybe a strobe light.

Focus is a survival mechanism. It's not about discipline, laziness, or simply getting the paperwork done. It's the ultimate gift from our ancestors—if we know how to activate it.

We didn't dominate the earth with an eight-hour workday or spread from continent to continent, crossing the vast oceans, by sitting in a cubicle. Instead, inspiration, creativity, and genius all happened in short moments when people activated this age-old focused burst of energy.

CHAPTER **SUMMARY**

- The brain covers for its mistakes. When trying to understand the brain, it turns out that we are terrible at monitoring our own ability. The brain seems to deceive itself, making us think we are focused or alert when we are not. This has also been observed with brain injuries and ailments like Alzheimer's. So, even if you think you're focused, forgetful, or smart—or not—you need objective tests to measure those things accurately.

- Humans get more focused, alert, and intelligent as they get closer to a deadline. It's like getting closer to a predator. It wakes us up and brings out talents we didn't know we had.

- Using our brain's flight or fight response, we can focus better in less time using the Focus-Burst Technique.

19 | Questions That Kill Focus

The Focus-Burst Technique works well, but I discovered a few mistakes that can destroy these gains.

There is a principle that states that we can only consciously think of one thing at a time. Yet, we also know that our brain processes information subconsciously during our down time. Focus bursts take advantage of both of these principles by forcing you to focus on one thing at a time in a very intense way, while also giving you the mental break to allow your subconscious mind to work on tougher problems in between times of action. Circus performers of the past and present have used this to block out pain. (I know this because I have met them! Being a Guinness Record holder means you will meet circus people at some point.)

One friend of mine did a trick that involved being run over by a pickup truck. He would lie down on stage with a ramp on either side of him and his very large, exposed belly sitting in between. The front tire would roll over him, followed by the back. Then he would stand up, seemingly unscathed.

There are a bunch of tricks like this involving a performer getting stabbed, poked, crushed, or otherwise put in pain for the entertainment of an audience. I will reveal how it's performed right here.

The trick is that there is no physical trick. What you see happens. There is no trick hand or hidden reinforcement armor. When the performer is run over by a truck, he is really rolled over—but smoothly in one motion, so it causes great pain but no permanent injury. So the only trick left is to deal with the pain. The real trick is a brainhack. At the exact second the truck is rolling over him, his mind focuses on a very compelling image. He didn't tell me what he imagines, but it's a very compelling scene that he loves to think about. Basically, a happy place. If it's timed just right, the brain moves to the happy place at the exact second the truck moves into position, and he does not feel a thing.

These performers do not last long, because they really are damaging their bodies. But, at least in the moment, they don't feel the pain.

A part of this is singularity of purpose. Before I decided to go for a world record, I was all over the place with my plans. I wanted to start a business, write a book, and even compete on game shows. Then, I had one conversation with Mr. Muller, the teacher who made the biggest impact on my life.

I was venting about how bad the system was for me, and how well I learned on my own with these techniques. His answer changed my life and knocked the chip off my shoulder.

"Prove it," he said.

He was kind, not malicious. He had seen me recall playing cards and knew I was onto something. But it was just a trick unless I did something big.

"If you can figure out your memory, David, and figure out how to read better than any dyslexic person I know," he continued, "then show them more. Keep building your system until it can do everything, and then teach others. These kids need all the help they can get, and teachers take many forms."

I was close to graduating high school at the time. I was doing well but had been angry over how things could have turned out differently. Mr. Muller took those blinders off and showed me I wasn't alone. Potentially great students were struggling, and good teachers were struggling to reach them.

I sheepishly told him about the idea of breaking a Guinness Record, and he smiled and encouraged me to do it. His encouragement made it go from a thought to a dream and a goal.

Get the Right Instructions

So, if a circus performer can block out conscious pain just by focusing on something else, then you can bet that it's impossible to think of more than one thing at a time, continuously. Our brains swap topics in and out of our consciousness like a game of musical chairs. One minute you can look at a TV, and the next at your phone, but you're not paying full attention to any one of them.

When we are given tasks, this can get even more difficult, because the biggest attention seeker in your brain is the brain itself. The first thing to consider to achieve effortless focus is the curious, questioning brain.

Let's say your boss gave you a task that seemed like busy work. But she left out some instructions. You had to organize a bunch of forms by the number at the top of the page, but there are two numbers at the top. How focused would you be? Not at all. Because your brain cannot start without knowing the answer to the question, "Which number do I use?"

Not only that, but not knowing why the forms need to be organized in the first place leaves a lot of questions. This is more than a minor annoyance, but a real loss of productivity. When I started hosting online classes, I discovered that my students were losing focus trying to work on tasks late at night but kept on getting caught up in minor snags like not knowing the word count for an assignment. The professors were surprised and skeptical, but they saw a big boost in performance after they habitually posted all the instructions for an assignment on their site. There was an uptick in quality, and more submissions came in earlier. Questions are so powerful that your brain prioritizes them. So much so that you can't truly focus on even part of a task as long as you have questions about the entire thing.

Hack focus by getting all the right instructions or having access to them before you start the work.

I could inspire others and maybe teach my system everywhere. Motivation is key to tackling a big task. Often, a challenge is much more difficult than it first appears. It always takes more effort and time to succeed at a goal than we think at first. That's why most people fail—not from lack of strategy or expertise, but simply by giving up. When I started to doubt, I would think of a happy place image, and that moment was a powerful one.

STIMULATION

Some people reading will fight me on the idea that we can't multitask. They like to have multiple screens on at the same time or have the TV on in the background as they read or study. I have been known to do the same thing. But if we look a little closer, we'll see that these examples only prove the point. They show another part of the brain focus mechanism: stimulation.

As you learned in the speed-reading chapter (page 73), the brain does not have any set level (like speed or temperature) that it runs on. It only compares current sensory input to similar past input. If you extend that to studying, the brain gets used to a specific level of stimulation (information coming at you in an interesting way or speed). If you dip below that level, your brain will tell you that it's bored and can't focus. The problem is that we then turn on the TV to get a little background noise and feel better—but tests show that once we do that, our performance suffers.

When you do any cognitive work, like studying or even watching a movie, you are geared to receive a specific level of stimulation. To understand this, try watching a movie from the 1960s or '70s and you will see what I mean. It could be a great movie, but if you are used to modern, fast-paced scenes and dialogue, it will feel like the movie is dragging by slowly.

Meditation can change this. When we meditate, it's like turning down the stimulation level of the brain. That can feel great too. After all, most people's goal on vacation is to slow down and relax. The question is not how much stimulation is good for the brain; that depends on the activity. Background entertainment is a double-edged sword, because you will score lower if you have it on but turning it off will only make you zone out.

There is a third solution, covered in the next chapter, that comes when you understand that the brain does not focus so you can pass a test. Focus is a survival mechanism.

CHAPTER **SUMMARY**

- Based on the fact that the brain can only focus on one thing at a time, performers with perfect timing are able to distract themselves so much they do not feel pain. The distraction is imagining a happy place. It's different for everyone, but it's so interesting to the brain that it takes you away from the pain in the moment.
- Get the right instructions. Sun Tzu said that if the general's orders aren't clear, it's the fault of the general. When instructions are missing or confusing, the brain compensates by asking questions. This distracts, and focus is lost.
- Hack stimulation! Learning can be boring, so our brain seeks stimulation and we turn on background noise. Don't do this. Instead, make what you are learning more intense, giving the brain the stimulation it needs.

20 | Focus on Guinness

Near the end of high school, I told my friends and family that I was planning to go for a Guinness Record for memorizing the order of fifty-two decks of cards. They thought I was crazy.

It would be a feat like none other. First, I could only see each card once. No repetition. The number of errors allowed was extremely low. When you recall items in memory competitions, a wrong answer just gets the point deducted. For this record, if I got more than 0.5% wrong, I would lose the whole record. That means out of the 2,704 cards I needed to recall for this record, I was allowed only 13 wrong answers. On top of that, the decks of cards would be shuffled all together, not in separate packs, which means I could not use the process of elimination to figure out a missing or forgotten link in each deck.

Also, my brain was playing tricks on me. I would imagine a card in my mind's eye, but then it would flip. I often turned a 7 into a J for Jack, making an error. Maybe that was related to my dyslexia.

Looking back, I should have tried to find an easier record. Turns out there were other memory records that were much easier that I didn't know about. But there is something about aiming at an impossible goal. If you don't give up, it changes you.

I took the first step by creating a new card code based on the visual list in Chapter 15, but this was more advanced because I could combine five cards into one mental image, cutting down on the number of links I needed to make.

The big challenge left was achieving the incredibly high level of accuracy needed for this record. I would need to have a hack that would prevent my brain from getting distracted.

As I started planning, it seemed that everyone suddenly came out of the woodwork with terrible advice. In my family, we used to have big gatherings that included extended family, cousins, related families, and their plus-ones. So, it was common for me to meet people I had never seen or would never see again.

At one of these gatherings, shortly after I graduated high school, I remember dealing with three people in a row pulling me aside, thinking their argument would convince me to stop. They made it their mission to stop me from trying to go for this record. It was the crab bucket (page 50) at work. It baffled me why anyone thought it was even their business in the first place. Interestingly, this conflict is the perfect place to explain the next focus principle: the concept that focus is about trusting your first thought.

THE TRAFFIC LIGHT METAPHOR

Imagine a thought experiment where you are at a busy intersection with the task of taking photos of expensive cars. For this, you have been given control over the traffic light and a camera that can focus on the car in the front of the line. All you can see in the line are old, beat-up, bad cars. What would be the best strategy to success?

Of course, at first you would activate the stoplight several times and probably curse out loud that there are so many beat-up, bad-looking cars. Pretty soon you would realize there is nothing to be gained holding back traffic, and you would let them go until you see some really pricey cars.

By now you should realize my metaphor is not about cars. This is a description of how the imagination works when trying to come up with creative ideas. The cars are your ideas, and you can't control their quality or how fast they come to you.

It's almost impossible to generate good ideas. Most great writers just generate a lot of ideas and select the good ones. But we often make the mistake of lamenting how bad our ideas are. That questioning of our own self is like hitting the stoplight, leaving the really good ideas waiting in traffic.

The only thing you have control over is stopping these ideas, so the best strategy for focus is to think without judging yourself. Let the ideas flow. You can still edit and be critical of whatever you are working on, just stop judging yourself. Get into a Zen frame of mind and let the thoughts flow so you don't become your own worst enemy.

Hack Creativity with Your First Thought

Trust your ideas. If you write, then get all your ideas out before editing. If you are planning, then go with your gut till the plan is made; then, and only then, critique it. Focus is a state of mind and critical thought gets in the way of a focused mind.

LIMITING BELIEFS ZAP FOCUS

This mindset of trying new things and experimenting ran right into the limiting beliefs of my extended family. I would not have succeeded if I had let them control my thoughts. See if this story reminds you of any limiting beliefs you've heard.

Some people felt they needed to try and stop me. Some thought I was trying a big practical joke. Others just wanted me to avoid embarrassment or disappointment, but the worst believed in a conspiracy.

The overall theme from the naysayers was that working-class people like me could never rise above their class because the 1% will stop them, or that the only way to succeed or make money is on the backs of others. I heard this nonsense so many times it became like background noise.

I found myself in a circle of lawn chairs, discussing this topic. I had shared my dream of starting a business to share my brainhacks, and several people were trying to dissuade me. They didn't think that aiming for financial success this way was an achievable goal. An older plus-one that I had never met before (or since) was very passionate about convincing me with his conspiracy theory. He said, "The 1% run the economy, and they won't loan money, give you sales, or allow others to work with you unless you do their bidding."

I explained I was aware of how some companies try to influence laws to stop small businesses from competing.

"You're so naïve, David. They rigged the system. The 1% changed the laws so workers can never get agency," he condescended. He continued, nodding at his own points. Finally, he revealed the source of his irrational hatred of the rich: anti-Semitism. "When people talk about the 1%, we're talking about those people who wear the little hats and go to the temple," he said.

A mix of disgust and shock overwhelmed me. Some in the group nodded in agreement. Others left the group horrified—me included.

I've been in the business world for thirty years now and personally, I know wealthy people from every walk of life, background, and religion. They are no different from people I have met at the bottom of the so-called hierarchy. In this man, the Crab Bucket mentality had been taken a step further—from bringing down individuals around him to spreading hate against entire groups of people. This perspective is far from harmless.

* * *

In your family, the story may be different, but the result is the same. Others' limiting beliefs can have negative effects, including lowering your motivation to succeed. You picked up this book for a reason. You want to achieve something beyond where you started. Just aiming higher and moving forward is something to be proud of. Don't let the Crab Bucket win.

Sometimes, working toward this Guinness Record made me feel like the world was against me. I really appreciate the few friends and relatives who supported me at the time. Aside from these people, that period was a sea of negativity for me. Two other relatives at the family gathering actually challenged me to a bet—they bet me $20 cash that I would fail.

I took the bet.

Full Focus-Burst Technique

1. **Get the Right Instructions and End Limiting Beliefs**
   When we receive confusing or incomplete instructions, our brain asks questions to fill in the blanks. But unfortunately, this halts the flow/focus state in its tracks.

2. **Zen: Trust Your First Thought**
   Second-guessing the brain creatively can cause the same kind of shutdown of flow state. It's best to let the ideas flow; get them out, then put on a different mindset to judge them.

3. **Timed Intervals:** Use timed intervals to focus. Break up your task into chunks and use the timer and the goal to raise the intensity of the task and awaken your peak potential.

CHAPTER **SUMMARY**

- You can hack your creativity by trusting your ideas and turning off your inner critic.
- Limiting beliefs from friends and family can interfere with your focus. The best technique in the world will not work if you don't think you can do it.
- With the Full Focus-Burst Technique, you get the right instructions and end limiting beliefs.

AXIOM NINE

THE STRESS IS NOT
THE STRESSOR

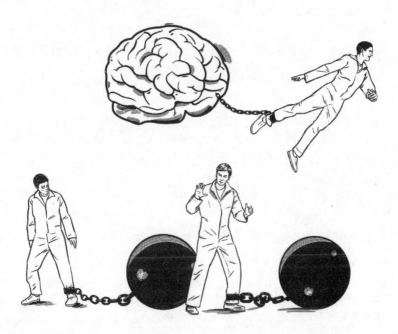

In science, a stressor is an external stimulus, like a job or a traffic jam. The term "stress" is used to define our reaction to these stimuli. Stress shortens life, lowers IQ, and feels terrible. It's a vestigial feature of our evolution that has not changed to meet the challenges of the modern world. To master life, we need to understand and take control of our stress reaction. More than any other factor of brain function, stress can be hacked.

21 | Stress, When Focus Thinks It's Going to Lose

In my last year of high school, and during my transition from school to starting and running my own business, I found this Full Focus-Burst Technique changed things significantly. For starters, I stopped procrastinating on projects—because it was easier to break the task up into bite-sized chunks and do them between breaks. I also found that the breaks became rewards. Instead of feeling guilty for watching my favorite TV shows, I used them to motivate me to keep going. I would record my favorite shows on VHS and then do focus bursts for hours while binge-watching them . . . seven minutes at a time. I honestly started to run out of things to do.

The best part was the lack of fatigue. Oddly—considering my disdain for higher education—my first few memory training jobs were to teach college students how to prepare for exams. When we did the Focus-Burst Technique properly, my students and I could study for hours at a time, and then just socialize feeling not the least bit tired. I didn't need coffee or pressure to be productive.

By doing focus bursts daily, I trained my brain to get into and out of the flow state at will. Today, I run three companies and have many employees and clients to keep track of. I do all the work I can in focus bursts, like going through email, doing administrative work, writing, working in sales, and even designing a robot prototype for a new tech startup called FarrowBOT. I've even written this book with focus bursts.

* * *

It was out of high school and still about six months away from breaking the Guinness Record when I started to use focus bursts to memorize cards, and I saw immediate results. I practiced the Focus-Burst Technique daily and did some trial runs that worked. Now was the time to find out how far I could push my brain.

As I mentioned in the previous chapter, I decided to attempt to memorize fifty-two decks of playing cards—2,704 cards in total—in order to break the Guinness Record. It was a target well above Dominic O'Brien's forty-deck record and had a poetic dimension, as I would be recalling as many decks of cards as there are cards in a deck.

I created a journey to link the cards to, just like you learned in Chapter 15. I wanted a journey that would keep me interested, so I moved from the real world into the sci-fi world. Instead of linking cards to lamps and tables, I used scenes from my favorite movies at the time. The entire *Star Wars* and *Indiana Jones* original trilogies worked well. I made a list of all the scenes and used them like rooms in the Journey Brainhack. I had cards being shot by Han Solo and other cards being force-choked by Darth Vader. That would keep me interested, I thought.

Finally, I needed the perfect venue—one that would give me the best chance of success. So, I looked for Guinness-related places and found the Guinness World Records Museum on Clifton Hill in Niagara Falls, Ontario. Unfortunately, it had no power to officially approve the record. Still, I thought it would have the greatest interest in hosting a Guinness Record.

I was right, and after a few phone calls, they arranged the time and place. I was plagued by negative thoughts from the Crab Bucket in my life. This hack made a difference. It's basically a memory technique for emotions.

Whenever I began to feel negative, this helped. I was ready to break a Guinness Record!

The Negative Redirect Hack

The problem with negative thoughts is that you can't stop thinking about them. They will not go away, and the harder you try to fight them, the more power they get. But you *can* redirect that energy to a positive thought.

Step One: Write down the images or scenarios you think of when you fall into a negative thought cycle. Think of all the phrases people say and all the worst-case scenarios.

Step Two: Imagine what the positive version of that situation would be. Change the image into a positive and believable version. Don't go from worst to best case. I find this works better if you go from the worst case to a believable positive interpretation of events. This path is easier to think of when you are in a panic.

Step Three: Link these two situations together so that one reminds you of the other. You can do this by imagining them happening like a movie in which you control the outcome. Repeat this process several times until this redirect is second nature. Like building muscles, this creates pathways that are stronger than your negative ones.

SHOW TIME

The museum itself was perfect for a spectacle. The front held several actual Guinness Records and recreations of past ones. There was a chair where the world's tallest man, Robert Wadlow, had sat; he was 8′11″. There were re-creations of the fattest twins riding motorcycles, and a giant, perfectly round rock sitting on a water fountain in the center of the walkway. The base's fountain pushed water up to suspend the rock slightly, allowing people to roll it with their hands.

The inside of the museum was much more distracting, though. Every inch was lined with record-breaking exhibits, and it was loud. I remember one interview from *That's Incredible!* (a show from the '80s) about a man who was going to ride the world's smallest bike. As he was mounting it, the announcer said, "From the sublime to the uncomfortable." This track played on a loop. I must have heard it a hundred times before my event began.

When I got to the museum, I got to work right away. The record required several witnesses with no connection to me and who were upstanding community members (Guinness rules, not mine). They started by shuffling fifty-two decks of playing cards all together into a big pile. There was a shuffle machine, and a few extra hands, to help. After shuffling all the cards into a random sequence, they sorted them back into packs of fifty-two to make handling easier, making sure to follow Guinness's existing rules for the record. (Niagara Falls is also a casino town, so playing cards were easy to find. More than one of the local casinos was curious about my card skills.)

Going into the event, I was doing great at first. My card code technique allowed me to memorize multiple cards for each link, and I used scenes from movies as my Journey Brainhack, placing card links all around scenes from my favorite movies at the time.

Every review I did in my mind had nothing missing or challenging. But, of course, no one had any idea how well things were going on the outside because I was just memorizing.

The museum owner used this as an opportunity to get publicity, and I had made the mistake of agreeing to do interviews before I was done memorizing. After several interviews, I lost my focus. I was rushing now to catch up, and I made mistakes in my links.

My perfect streak of focus was derailed, and I knew I was sunk. I missed a couple of links in a review of deck thirty-four; then, it got worse. I panicked and missed sequences I had already committed to memory. I lost focus and, with it, my confidence. As a result, in the last few decks, I made even more mistakes. In all my training, I didn't consider that focus can turn to panic very quickly.

I tried to shake my head and walk it off. But, instead, I recalled the cards I did well at first again and even recalled some parts I thought I had completely blanked on. But as I went in further, I added up more and more mistakes, ultimately missing more cards than were allowed for the record. Looking back, I did a fantastic job considering it was my first try. My rate of mistakes was only about 2%. But that's a far cry from the 0.5% allowed for the record. I had failed.

The media ran the story of my trial and failure. I was Icarus incarnate. The toughest part was going back home and speaking to every person who told me I couldn't succeed. Of course, they all had the courtesy to find me and say, "I told you so." But I still had the supporters in my corner. I told the owner of the museum that I was going to come back and break the record, but he said no. He told me I had one shot, and it was over. That was tough to hear.

Oddly, a sense of calm came over me after the event was done. The stress was off. After having done the event and failed, I knew that it couldn't get any worse, and honestly, this wasn't that bad. Fear of failure was just an illusion. The tiger had gotten a hold of me and ripped me to pieces, and I was still here. And now I knew for sure how to break the record. I needed to understand the role of stress. To fight stress, I used event rehearsal.

I would go through the image of succeeding several times every morning and evening. Eventually it was second nature, and I had confidence that

Event Rehearsal

This is a powerful tool used by everyone from Olympic athletes to samurai to award-winning rock stars. The idea is simple. When you visualize something, the brain thinks that it has actually happened, because your visualization travels through the same pathways in the brain that sensory information does. Knowing this, sit down and visualize your event, from beginning to end, going perfectly.

Visualization is not as powerful as an experience in the real world of course, so to make this work, imagine it over and over. It helps to do it in super-fast forward.

I would succeed the next time. If I didn't go back and try again, they would forever know me as the guy who failed. To bring a win from this defeat, I would have to master stress as I did focus.

The relatives who bet $20 that I would fail came around to ask for their money. Instead of handing it over, I grinned and said, "How about double or nothing?"

CHAPTER **SUMMARY**

- Like mental aikido, you can take negative comments, thoughts, and limiting beliefs and redirect them for your benefit. Just identify the messages you don't like and make a memory link to remind you of a positive counter. Today, every time I hear that only a small percentage of ADHD kids succeed, I think I must be in that percent—and that with training those kids could become the majority. This redirect kept me going through the negativity of well-meaning people.
- Event rehearsal is the secret tool of many performers and athletes. On some level, the brain thinks something you imagine actually happens. By imagining over and over an event going the way you want it to, you build up a level of confidence as if you had actually done the event, even if it's your first time.

22 | If at First You Don't Succeed

> When everything seems to be going against you, remember
> that the airplane takes off against the wind, not with it.
>
> **—Henry Ford**

L et's go back to our idea of the hunter-gatherer looking at a tiger, spear
in hand, hunters to the right and left. Ready for the fight. What happens
if, just then, he twists his ankle and, while falling over, breaks his spear?
The tiger roars, and his friends run away, leaving him stuck with a broken
stick against the world's most fearsome predator. Confidence turns to fear,
and his focus shifts to stress.

Stress and panic, like any other response, exist to help you. However,
in this case, it's saved for the worst-case scenario. When the hope of survival is unlikely, the brain changes strategy and the body prepares to be
damaged. After the epinephrine from your focus session wears off, con-
tinuing to try to focus and push yourself is like telling the brain you are
in danger.

Nature thinks that if you survive, you will be injured and bleeding,
maybe with broken bones or worse.

With this in mind, it's obvious how living in a state of constant stress
is killing us. Something called the hypothalamic-pituitary-adrenal (HPA)

axis sends a series of signals through the brain and body that ends up releasing cortisol, the stress hormone. Not only is cortisol an anti-inflammatory painkiller (like Advil, but much stronger), but it also interferes with focus. If focus is the body's way of preparing for a fight-or-flight situation, then the full stress response is your body's way of preparing for losing that fight. You learned in the previous chapter how small amounts of stress can focus the brain. This is true, but brain chemistry is all about intensity. Like taking medication, for instance: a little bit can heal but too much can overdose. The problem is our brains never evolved to handle most of the modern challenges we face every day, so they tend to overreact, causing more problems. We stress about our job or the rent, making our bodies prepare for a fight that could include wounds and blood loss. But that fight never comes, so the stress never goes.

Most modern humans live as if there is a tiger in their midst every day. Unfortunately, this hypervigilance has the added consequence of building up our overall stress levels, making it harder and harder to relax the longer we live in high stress (similar to how it's harder to lose weight once you develop insulin resistance). A mental task like studying or test-taking can quickly turn from focus to stress for this reason because you have trained your brain to do that already. Both exist on a spectrum. So, when mastering focus, we need to master the stress response and how to hack it.

MASTERING THE STRESS RESPONSE

The hack for stress is to understand that it is just a reaction. A specific reaction geared toward handling predators in the wild. By rationalizing the stress, we can understand it and start to prevent the stress response in the first place.

Learning that you have power over your stress reactions is important, but if you deal with anxiety or phobias, you may not feel like you have much control. The first thing I discovered is that stress is stupid. Literally, stress is a function of the primitive brain. When it takes over (a process called amygdala hijacking), it completely bypasses the cerebral cortex. It returns your brain to a primitive state.

Let's look back at our evolutionary past before we had the cerebral cortex (the higher level of the brain, the part with all the wrinkles). There was our limbic brain, the more primitive part underneath. Before humans walked the earth, the limbic brain did the thinking, and it was very basic. Often called the lizard brain, the amygdala doesn't think as much as it reacts to environmental stimuli. This happens to be a very good thing when the world is full of angry predators that want to kill and eat humans. But in the modern world, this mechanism reacts to everything from the rent being due to people disliking us on social media. So, our stress is like a caveman part of us constantly being scared by the environment. And when it gets scared, it takes over.

The lizard brain is connected to the thinking brain through nerves (information pathways), but more pathways are coming from it than going to it. This is why it has so much control over you when you panic, but you have very little influence on it. That's why you will never think or self-talk your way out of stress. There is simply no pathway to reach it using that method. In my case, stress isn't just unhealthy—it will sink me. This is because cortisol, the stress hormone, directly interferes with the brain's ability to form and recall memories. Not to mention that anything close to a stress response starts to shut down the higher brain functions for the sake of survival.

Like it or not, evolution has concluded that you don't need to be smart when fighting for your life. But there are some simple ways to hack stress and hopefully turn this scary wild animal into your pet.

The best success image I remembered was an experience I had playing football in junior high school. Being athletic helped keep me healthy and lowered my chronic pain flare-ups (though I did still have some pain days where I needed to skip practice).

I played the guard position, and my entire job was basically to line up in front of another person and hit the guy in front of me as hard as possible. If they got past me, it only took two steps to reach the quarterback.

Success Image Hack

One tool to keep focused and positive is the Success Image Technique. This is similar to the idea of the happy place image (page 129), but instead of taking you away from a stressful moment, it makes you feel strong and confident to handle the moment. It's a way to tap into powerful experiences from your past.

Step One: Search your memory for times when you felt strong or unbeatable. These are often rare situations, and not the cliche times when you graduate or win something. They're points that marked a massive change in your life.

Step Two: Make the image clear by visualizing the story before and after it to reinforce the feeling of greatness.

Step Three: Practice bringing it up when you start to feel stressed. Either link it to the situation you dread or make a habit of going to this image when you want a confidence boost. Powerful emotional situations can interrupt the pattern of stress and shock you out of fear and panic.

The successful image you choose doesn't have to have anything to do with the event you are trying to go after. It just needs to make you feel powerful. For example, the image I used for my second Guinness attempt was a memory of a sports event.

One game, I was squaring off against a guy who was at least fifty pounds heavier than me and a foot taller. We were both in junior high at the time, but he had facial hair. I honestly remember asking if he was allowed to have so much facial hair because he was clearly older than everyone else. As a result, I coined the nickname Blackbeard for him. For the entire game, there were two major hits I felt every time they snapped the ball: him hitting me and me hitting the ground. I was getting my butt kicked.

Late in the game, my team found ourselves close to the end zone, and the coach called a running play. That meant I was supposed to push over the guy in front of me and give enough room for the QB to run past me to score a touchdown. For the first time, I questioned the coach's sanity because there was no way I could move the guy in front of me. I reminded the coach about his illegal amount of facial hair and everything, but it was no use. The play was going to happen.

Sun Tzu said that a small force can defeat a larger one if they are in "death ground." When you place your army in an impossible situation, with their back against a mountain or wall and with no hope of survival except winning, they will fight like lions. It was time to see if that was true.

Blackbeard chuckled at me with the confidence of a man who had won every encounter. I cleared my head, shook off all the bruises and hits from that day, and gathered all the energy I had. Balling my hands into tight fists, I waited on the heels of my feet. The ball snapped, and I stayed low, trying to get under him. Throwing both fists up just under his ribcage, I heard the wind escape his lungs all at once. My shoulders followed the fists, lifting him and flipping him over like a pancake. Just as the quarterback flew past me to the left, I felt the ground shake when he landed flat on his back. I didn't see the QB score. The game faded into a blur, and it was just me, staring down at Blackbeard's face, which was painted with shock and disbelief.

That face was my image of success. Whenever I doubted myself or felt like I was getting stressed, I thought of old Blackbeard and felt powerful again.

* * *

When I was twenty-one, I felt ready for another shot at the Guinness. I called up the media contacts I had from the last attempt to break the card memorizing record to tell them I planned to try again. They were excited about a comeback story and said they would cover it again. However, I told them that this time, to avoid getting distracted, I had to hold off on interviews until after I got the record.

Then, I called up the Guinness Museum, asking to return to try again at the record in a few weeks. They refused, reminding me they were not in the habit of performing record attempts. I paused for a second, but my stress hacks kicked in as I thought of Blackbeard, and something in me got a little cocky.

I told them that several reporters were going to show up in a few weeks asking about the memory guy attempting to break a record again, and he would have to tell them that I was told not to try. Afraid of the bad press, he agreed to let me try one more time. As I hung up, I realized I had legit just blackmailed a guy into letting me try again. I had raised the stakes even higher than before. The pressure was on.

The day of the event was exhausting. Nevertheless, I did the event as planned, taking nearly eight hours just to recall the cards alone. I was numb. Logically, I knew I broke the record. My family arrived, and the museum owner paid for all of us to go to a restaurant. He went from hating me for blackmailing him into respecting me for it—even bragging about it. The reporters swarmed me, and I did several interviews in a row, talking about my experience. By the end of the day, I was exhausted—absolutely drained. With a splitting headache, I crashed at the motel beside the museum for a few hours.

In the morning, a phone call from *Fox* woke me up. I was just getting out of my sleepy haze and answered the phone with the words, "From the sublime to the uncomfortable," just like I had heard again and again in the museum before both my record-breaking attempts, much to the confusion of the interviewer. I crashed again, returning to my Odinsleep. Later that day, just past noon, I woke up, headache gone, feeling refreshed. More than that, I was positively giddy. It was a sunny afternoon, near the beginning of the tourist season in Niagara Falls, so the mostly empty motel was being prepared to welcome guests.

I remember there were these rectangular flower boxes that hung off the balcony of the motel. As my girlfriend pulled back the curtain and rolled open the glass door to reveal the balcony, I saw they had filled the boxes with small red flowers that morning. I said to myself curiously, "Those flowers weren't there yesterday." Then, it fully hit me what had happened the day before. In a snap, all the stress was gone, and the feeling of success finally consumed me. I said out loud, smiling, "And I didn't have a Guinness record yesterday either!"

From that moment on, those flowers replaced Blackbeard as my success image.

I still needed to wait months to get the official approval from *The Guinness Book of Records*. Hours of footage and witness signatures, all strictly adhering to established rules, needed to be sent in. But the media had already declared it a success, and I was riding high. I got to go back to all the people who said I would never succeed and finally be the one who said "I told you so." To this day, no one remembers that I failed the first time. And for the record, I still am waiting to collect the $80 from those bets.

RIP MR. MULLER

Lives change, split, and grow like tree branches. Why did that branch curve right instead of left? DNA? An obstacle? Or was it following the sun? The beauty of this tree, unique among the forest because of a thousand decisions lost to time.

—D.F.

Years later, the memory club, school events, and Guinness Record attempts were a thing of the past, and I was doing well in my career as a memory expert. One day, Mr. Muller contacted me, and my excitement to hear from him quickly turned to dread.

He had a terminal diagnosis and had been given weeks to live. This man was beloved by all—a mentor not just to me but also to most of the kids I grew up with. He had taught and influenced thousands of students, but he was calling me.

He said his dying wish was to have me pass on my memory techniques to his grandkids. "I want to give them the gift of memory because I want them to remember me, and I can't imagine anything else I could show them that would have a bigger impact on them growing up," he said.

This was and remains the greatest honor of my entire life. But I was also nervous, because teaching kids can be hit-or-miss, and failure terrified me. But it was his dying wish. So, I dropped everything and went to his family. My goal was to teach them the basics—memorizing some playing cards. I sat down and made games out of practice. We went over the visual card list, and I got them to draw right on the cards to make the images their own. It only took a few days, and they were ready to show Grandpa. I'll never forget the sound of joy in his voice when he called me to thank me.

Shortly after that, he passed away.

I got to the funeral just as the service was starting. The church, St. Matthew's, was packed—standing room only. I saw students of all ages lining the walls while passionate family members and fellow teachers spoke at the front. He was a founder of the Art Package Program and defended the power of education and the arts to change lives. Based on the attendance and the tears in the audience, he had changed all the students' lives that he touched. When people ask me what it takes to be a good teacher in an interview, I think of him and of that day.

During the eulogy, they mentioned me, and used Mr. Muller's wish to bring the gift of memory to others as an example of his commitment to education as an agent of change. They called me world-famous. I was embarrassed, not feeling worthy of the honor. This man had given me so much.

I still felt in his debt.

By giving the gift of memory to you, dear reader, I hope I can start to pay back that debt.

CHAPTER **SUMMARY**

- The first step to getting rid of a problem is to be aware of it. So the best anti-stress hack is to be aware of the science behind what is causing the stress. Realize that it's just a leftover tool of evolution, and you do not need to react this way. This is easier said than done, and that is why using the other stress hacks are useful. But they won't work unless you know how stress works first.

- With the Success Image Hack, think of a situation that still makes you feel good, strong, or even powerful. There are moments in our lives that stick out. Choose the climax of one such event and hold onto the image clearly anytime you start to panic.

AXIOM TEN

SUB-WORDS

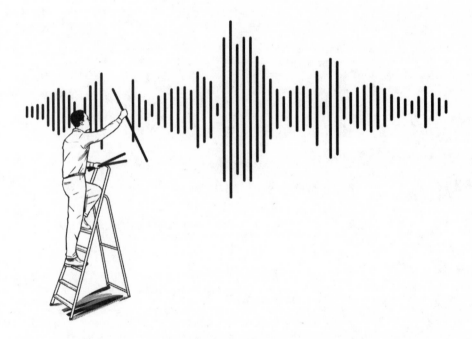

We can link up numbers and objects, symbols and concepts, but complex words have been beyond us, until now. A foreign word or technical term is just a set of sounds. Play with the syllables in your mind's ear until you hear something familiar. Then substitute the new item for the difficult word.

23 | Hack Languages

This chapter and the next are the story of how I memorized 1,400 words of Cantonese in one weekend . . . and then immediately regretted it.

In my twenties, I lived in Toronto. It wasn't perfect, but it's hard to deny the multicultural success of the city itself. At some point, Toronto had the world's second-largest population of expats from a variety of nations including Tibet, Sri Lanka, Senegal, and more. In Toronto alone, Chinatown is the size of a real town. Toronto is also host to Caribana, the second largest Caribbean festival in the world—consider how absurd it is that this distinction belongs not to a city in the Caribbean but rather a city covered in snow half the year.

One exciting subgroup in Toronto is the large population of Cantonese speakers. Cantonese is a dialect of Chinese and is spoken in Hong Kong and the south of China. In the early days of China's communist crackdowns, Canada took in many Chinese refugees, who mostly settled in a small area of Toronto (called Chinatown today). It's about a block away from where I lived, and when walking in my neighborhood, I was just as likely to hear Cantonese as English. So what does a memory expert do in this case? He learns.

It helped that I was dating a woman whose family spoke Cantonese. Remember the movie *Lost in Translation*, where Bill Murray felt alone while surrounded by others because of the language barrier? I felt that daily.

Toronto has so many cultures and languages that I realized I would always be out of the loop (and the butt of a joke) if I didn't learn more. I would constantly encounter situations where I would walk into a room and people would switch from English to another language and continue talking. Their sideways glances made me feel like they were talking about me, but that had to be paranoia, right? It wasn't meant to be sinister. I'm sure they were friendly people, but it really threw off my confidence. So, I decided I would learn the language. I *am* the memory expert, right? So, how hard could it be?

My first step was to make a brain box.

The Brain Box Hack

I didn't invent the concept, but I recommend it to anyone having to learn a great deal of information.

Step One: You will need a box with five or six sections in it. Each section will be like a step in a ladder of memory. I took a shoebox and some duct tape to make my sections.

Step Two: Turn your vocabulary into flashcards. You may need to order a set or print them out.

Step Three: Play the brain box game. Take your flashcards and go through them one at a time, testing yourself to see if you recall them. Any you get right will be moved up to the second level of your box. Repeat the process when done with the second level, and winners graduate to the third and so on until they reach the end and leave the game. One mistake drops a word back down to one, though.

Step Four: Keep up this game until you have weeded out the easy vocab items. This can cut your work in half or more.

Step Five: Use memory techniques on the rest of the words and keep testing yourself until you're done.

This Brain Box hack is a serious timesaver, but I was in for a huge surprise. If language learning were a video game, French would be level 1, German or Russian would be level 5, and Cantonese or Thai would be level 200 at the far end of the game with the impossible big boss you can only defeat with cheat codes. Of course, my cheat codes were memory techniques, but that didn't mean it would be easy. I started looking at the vocabulary and getting the Internet to say words to me, but it was slow-going.

With my hearing problem and the complexity of the language, I needed more details. So, I signed up for a local class on Cantonese, and it started to click. It was not enough to connect words, though; I needed to understand the pronunciation and connect the right *tone* to the right word.

Here's what I mean. When you see a foreign word on the page, the mind sounds it out in our mother tongue. That's nearly always wrong. Even languages that have the same alphabet have different pronunciations. Growing up in Canada, everyone gets some instruction in French, but almost everyone butchers the accent. I still remember everyone laughing when someone in my French class said "What the seal?" because of how close the French word for seal sounds to an English swear word.

But in Cantonese, a word will change depending on the intonation used. Say the same word but raise your voice (a tone called "low rising"), and it means one thing; lower your voice ("high falling"), and it means something else.

The word *yut*, for example. Said one way, it means "January," and said another way, it means "each." Yet another tone makes it the word "one." In class, my teacher showed me these tones, but the whole process discouraged me. I was used to skills falling to my learning powers easily. I had already picked up a ton of vocabulary from other languages in my travels, but most weren't this difficult.

* * *

One day, I had a dinner date with my girlfriend's family. My girlfriend was having a heated conversation with her mother. They would argue, then smile at me and ask if I wanted more food. Then, I caught it. The tones and pronunciation allowed me to catch a familiar word for one brief second, and it sent a chill down my spine. I saw and heard the word *boyfriend*. Okay, they were talking about me, and I had to know what they were saying. I didn't have time to go through all the months of slow lessons in my class. I needed to jump ahead.

Memory techniques are often used by adults learning a second language. It's a huge advantage. With the proper technique, a person can commit to memory hundreds of vocabulary words in a day and remember them for as long as they want. To master a language, though, it's still necessary to practice making sentences and communicating, thinking, and even dreaming in the language. But having a tool like this to memorize vocabulary quickly gets students to understand in days what normally takes years to achieve.

That weekend, I memorized all the vocab in the language book I had—about 1,400 words.

CHAPTER **SUMMARY**

- When trying to memorize a large amount of technical or foreign terms, there is a simple shortcut to cut down on the amount of work that's needed. Make a box with about six compartments and turn your terms into flashcards. Then test yourself by going through them all. The ones you guess right go up in the box and the failures stay. After a few tests you can weed out the terms you already know, leaving behind your homework.

24 | Now You're Speakin' My Language!

The technique for memorizing foreign vocabulary and even things like technical or scientific terms is called substitute words. This is an age-old practice some believe dates back as far as Socrates.

> You can remember any new piece of information if it is associated to something you already know or remember.
>
> **—Attributed to Socrates by Harry Lorayne,**
> ***The Memory Book***

Substitute Words Brainhack

Note: All the complex and foreign words in this book have been romanized. That means they are spelled using the Latin alphabet with tones added.

To memorize a foreign word, we need to connect it to the English word that we already know or remember.

> **Step One:** Take the word you want to memorize and sound it out.
>
> **Step Two:** Play with how it sounds, and try to find words you know within the foreign word. Things that rhyme or sound similar are the words that will substitute for the foreign word in our memory link.
>
> **Step Three:** Make an image out of the result that is connected to the translation—the stranger the image, the better.

(The substitute word hack takes advantage of how a word sounds similar to another word. If you need to memorize how something is spelled, that is a different hack. For now, we'll focus on the sound.)

MEMORIZE THE SOUND

The first word I learned using this technique was *fenster*. It means "window" in German. I took a moment and imagined a fence over a broken window to my right and a crazy guy on the other side with a spoon rattling against the fence as if he is trying to stir it. Don't ask me why the image is so creepy, but it works.

How to Say "Hello" in Other Languages

Let's go through a few other examples:

Hello in Chinese is *ni hao (sounds like: Knee How)*: Imagine greeting someone in China, but as you step forward you trip and fall. Landing on your knee saying "OW" loudly. My Knee OW!! That's how I remember to say *ni* (sounds like "knee") *hao* (sounds like "how").

Hello in Arabic is *marhaba* (sounds like Mar-A-Bar to me): I imagine getting off a plane in Dubai and handing out Mars candy bars. Everyone who said hello, I said *marhaba* (sounds like "Mars bar"). Try it.

Hello in Mongolian is *saim bainoo* (Sounded to me like Salmon-No): I imagine a Mongolian waiter offering me a salmon dinner and I refuse. This is hilarious to me because salmon is one of my favorite foods.

Hello in Czech is *dobrý den,* so I imagine I'm standing at the Czech border with a guard holding back several Doberman dogs that want to attack me. *Dobrý den* sounds like Doberman.

Hello in Tibetan is *tashi delek.* Imagine the Dalai Lama needs a sandwich in a hurry, so he goes to the deli that makes the fastest sandwiches named after how you can dash in and dash out, the *tashi delek* ("dash-y deli").

Hello in Thai is *sawasdee* (sounds like Swat-Dee): If you are female, you end every sentence with *kha.* If you are male, you use *khrap.* So I imagine being pulled over by a cop and swatting at him to remember *sawasdee* ("swat") *khrap* ("cop") means hello. Seriously though, don't swat at a Thai cop. They will mess you up.

* * *

The Brain Box Hack (page 160) combined with Focus Bursts (page 124) and the Substitute Words Brainhack (page 163) helped me breeze through the vocab. As I said, in one weekend I had memorized over 1,400 Cantonese words.

There is, however, a difference between being able to recall vocab when tested and actually decoding a conversation. For fun, I would watch Hong Kong news (in Cantonese). I wasn't fluent, but I caught enough to follow along. Two weeks later, I sat down with my girlfriend, a few other friends, and her mom again ready to impress. It was a big function, and everyone was speaking loudly. At first, their words came so fast that I couldn't keep up. I had to think faster. The words were flying so quickly that I didn't have time to recall any links that I made in my apartment. But then something clicked. I understood. One conversation was about college, and another person talked about how they had bought a condo as an investment.

It wasn't all nice. I heard a guy say something rude about his white girlfriend while she was sitting right beside him. Then, I started to follow a conversation with my girlfriend's mother, and I instantly regretted it. I began to understand the conversation and why my girlfriend felt stressed around her mom. I was still new to the language, so I could only catch about half of the conversation, but plenty of repetition helped.

According to the mother, my girlfriend's sister had married a white guy and brought shame to their family. Her being with me was going to make it impossible to pass on their Chinese genes properly. She talked about keeping the race pure and I zoned out. I had learned so much of the language . . . but maybe I'd learned too much. On the other hand, I now knew enough to understand that my girlfriend's family would never accept me. If only I could have just stopped after learning the word *boyfriend*, I could have enjoyed being ignorant a little longer.

We broke up shortly after, and to be honest, we weren't a perfect fit for each other in many other ways. Looking back, I don't think we would have ever lasted, but something did change for me after that day. A year later, I was in an elevator going up to the top floor of a major law firm in Toronto. I was going to file for a patent in nanotech.

I was there because my dive into Cantonese had sparked my interest in using my memory skills to learn even more. I dove into languages, memorizing for fun, and this led to learning about technology. I became an expert on nanotech, even speaking at conferences and working as a design engineer, and today I have set my sights on a robotics startup called FarrowBOT. I never would have maxed out my learning stats like this if I didn't see what was possible by learning all that vocab so fast.

Two women entered the elevator speaking Mandarin. I was not as fluent in Mandarin as Cantonese, but like many language learners, I learned the dirty words first. So, when they started speaking, I recognized a lot. Thankfully when people speak about you in another language, they talk loudly, so I could hear clearly. Then, one of them said something about me that I won't repeat. Her friend joked back. This went on until we reached my floor.

Before I walked out, I thanked the woman for her compliment in Mandarin, and both of their jaws dropped. First, a look of terror went across their faces. Then, I smiled, and they started laughing and carrying on again as the doors closed.

CHAPTER **SUMMARY**

- One technique for memorizing foreign vocabulary is called substitute words. What we do is connect the word we want to learn to the English word that we already know. Take the word you want to memorize and sound it out. Using how the word sounds, find words you already know within the foreign word. Then, make an image out of what you came up with.

25 | Overnight Expert

Most conversations around education debate what system would be the best while putting all responsibility on teachers and the system to improve. I used to think that way too, but now my response is, "Then what?"

Someday, that student will be an adult who needs to learn the latest software program or industry info and be on their own with no system to help them. That's why every person needs to understand their brain and be able to teach themselves.

THE FUTURE IS SELF-TAUGHT

I was asked to speak at eBay in Silicon Valley as part of their speaker series. It was a great honor, but I was nervous to tell the audience that I was self-taught when it came to brain science. My knowledge, although extensive enough to author a study and work with neuroscientists as peers, is self-taught based on real-life application of brain science. Many of the concepts I teach, in fact, I invented.

When I told them about my lack of formal training in neuroscience but how my passion led to an autodidactic approach, I was treated with a standing ovation. My guide and close friend, Sergio Gonzalez, then head of innovation at eBay, explained, "There is a movement in Silicon Valley that is turning away from valuing traditional education. Google,

Facebook, and Apple have all dropped education requirements from their hiring practices. The reason is that the best programmers have no formal education." The self-taught hackers were outperforming the university computer science grads.

"How do they hire, then?" I asked, curious.

"They hold these big hiring competitions with hundreds of wannabe employees and show them a formula on a big screen. They have a certain amount of time to write a program to solve it. Those who fail leave and those who pass get the next more difficult puzzle, until only a handful of people are left. Almost every time, it's the high school grad hackers that remain, not the college grads."

There are mohawk-wearing, tattoo-covered programmers with no more than a high school education driving million-dollar cars and making your next phone because they are the best.

The best open-source projects like Tor and Firefox are run on an evolutionary basis where multiple programmers submit code and the ones that work are accepted and used. Even the world of biology has a self-taught group of biohackers slicing DNA in garages around the world that could lead to the next big thing.

Grand ideas have humble origins. Someday, we may compare this era to the Renaissance, when groups of self-directed learners like Leonardo da Vinci changed everything, paving the way for a better tomorrow.

MEMORY, NANOTECH, AND ROBOTS

From 2004 to 2007, I dove into the world of nanotechnology and became a self-taught expert. It was perfect for me. I was passionate about a new technology, but it was so unique that no one was truly an expert yet. After applying my memory techniques to languages with great success, I was hooked. I wanted to use this skill to get into tech the same way my dad did: learning by working on projects. Learning a new skill is just like learning a new language. There is culture, history, and more, but it all starts with just understanding the words for things.

Hacking Technical Skills

Step One: Plan your time. Put together a calendar to plan when you will study. I like having a focused burst session first thing in the morning to wake myself up.

Step Two: Set goals. It's important to stay motivated. Plan out your months with an end in mind. For example, I wanted to master nanotech and robotics to work in the field.

Step Three: Speed-read materials and pick out facts. As you consume the material, you will come across important definitions or descriptions of technical processes. When you want to memorize one of these things, make a list of these points and commit them to memory using focus bursts and memory techniques.

Step Four: Organize your information. We talked about using the Journey Brainhack to organize information. This is useful to keep track of lists. But organizing information can be a bigger task with more complex information.

It also helps to have the right support in your life. I had a new girlfriend who seemed to get me. I remember the day I told my then-girlfriend, now-wife, Andrea Zakel, about my plans.

"Of course you're going into nanotech," she said. "That makes perfect sense."

"Really? I thought this would come out of left field for you," I replied curiously.

"Oh, that's true too," she said between laughs. "But nothing about you surprises me anymore, Dave. If you want to do something, you don't follow a preset path that society tells us is the way things work. Instead, you just jump in and do the thing, so nanotech makes as much sense as anything else you do."

It was so refreshing to find a partner who understood me.

If I wanted to jump into a new field, I would have to learn the basics, but there were no textbooks on the subject. But there were patents—all freely available online. So, I dove into the new patents in this field. There were only a few hundred when I started.

Memorization Hack

When I found a term I didn't understand, I would memorize it. Here is one of my favorite examples because it seems so difficult to memorize at first; then, with the proper technique, it becomes child's play.

Excimer laser: An ultraviolet pulse laser that uses a combination of inert (noble) gases like krypton and xenon and reactive gases like chlorine and fluorine. It's used in eye surgery and the production of semiconductors.

Step One: Look at the definition and pick out the keywords from the entire term. You don't need to memorize *that* or *the*. Instead, just memorize the words that carry relevant meaning.

Step Two: Turn these highlighted words into substitute words. *Excimer* becomes *egg steamer* or maybe *eczema*; *krypton* becomes *Superman*; and *xenon* becomes *Xena*.

Step Three: Take a moment and make a fun story out of these components. I imagined Xena (the warrior princess) throwing Superman through the floor (fluorine).

I made a schedule to speed-read through them for about an hour or two a day. This allowed me to cover a couple hundred per week. While I was reading, more patents were approved because the field was expanding quickly. By the time a month had gone by, I had consumed over a thousand patents. I knew the basic terminology of several nanotech subfields. My favorite was microfluidics, a promising niche that used small amounts of fluid inside a set of channels to perform medical functions.

INFORMATION ARCHITECTURE

When learning a new field, we need to learn more than the individual terms. There is a knowledge base required to connect those terms to each other, forming a type of architecture.

All information takes a shape of some kind. Therefore, when memorizing information, it's useful to organize the data according to how the subject's internal structure works. For example:

- Lists are like chains linking one bit of information to another.
- Vocabulary words are best thought of in groups, such as groups of verbs or words for telling time.
- When mapped out, most technical subjects look like a root system. They start with the main subject, and then break into smaller parts until you get to the fine details.

Nanotech had a root system architecture. This is the shape of most hard academic subjects.

For example, if you studied law in school and charted out the connections between all the information, it would look like the root system of a tree with federal laws at the top that splits into criminal law, civil law, family law, etc. Then, each of those sections would be broken into subsections, eventually being reduced to the finest of details.

I was fascinated by how fluid flowed inside a small lab on a microfluidic chip, as it was called. I ended up starting a company to pursue a patent for an invention, which led me to speak at several nanotech conferences, and I even spoke to the President's task force on nanotech at the time. And I was on the path to launch the IP (intellectual property) for my invention. All this by being self-taught in the field.

However, nanotech turned out to be a bit of a bubble and didn't emerge as a field on its own. It was broken up into thousands of different areas and used in several different industries. The industry's volatile nature led the patent office to abruptly restrict the patents it was going to issue. So, my patent didn't get approved. But the experience I gained led me to more

---

Mapping Brainhack

When learning a new subject, it helps to map out these connections between sections spatially to learn the concepts better.

Step One: Make a chart of the big concepts, and then break them down to smaller sections.

Step Two: Apply the Journey Brainhack, and use a room or location for each section. This gives you an advantage on tests because there's a lot of information in subjects that sound similar. For example, science and law use Greek and Latin as a base for technical terms; thus, a concept in one area can sound very similar to a title in another.

Teachers know this and often make tests specifically to try and confuse the students. The idea is that if you know the material very well, you won't make a mistake. But if you map out the sections and organize them into different rooms, you can't be fooled. Even concepts that sound similar will feel far apart.

---

work in tech. I used my 3D modeling microfluidic skills in the medical device design field and expanded into robotics.

My most recent company is FarrowBOT Inc., a startup launching in 2022 that offers low-cost animatronic mannequins for retail and event spaces. For several years, I have enjoyed building the prototype, and now I get to fulfill my dream of being the CEO founder of a tech startup. All because of brainhacks.

CHAPTER **SUMMARY**

- Learning a technical subject involves several steps, from goal setting to planning your time. A good strategy is to use a combination of speed-reading to get a basic understanding of a subject and memory techniques to link together the information.

- Pick out key words and find substitute words for them. Then make a powerful set of memory links involving those words.

- As you progress through the subject, the act of organizing all this information will become its own challenge, so writing down the shape of the information helps to understand it better. When creating hundreds of memory links, it also helps to group them into journeys and rooms dedicated to specific sections.

AXIOM ELEVEN
DECODING

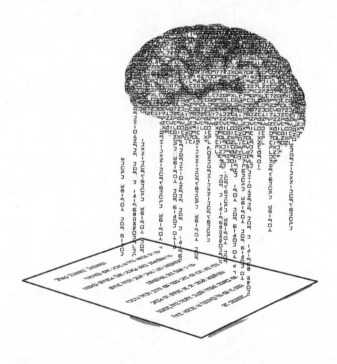

Beyond hacking your brain is the world of decoding others' brains. Our brains send messages to each other that most miss. Body language, lipreading, and lie detection are just a few hacks that make you feel like you can see into the minds of others, or at least sometimes glean the truth about those around you.

The world is talking to you in code. A brainhacker is a master decoder.

26 | Lipreading, Super Hearing with Your Eyes

I think you're on to something when you say you need a new way to learn," my mom told me as we walked through the door. "But I don't have all the answers, and sometimes teachers sure as hell don't know what to do with you." This was very early on in my brainhack journey—I must have been in elementary school—and my mom had taken me to the library. "You just need to figure out how that brain of yours works, and here is where you start," she said, gesturing to the walls of books.

I remember taking it all in and getting excited. She was right, of course—the library is an incredibly crucial source of learning. In the years since then, I've come to appreciate it more and more.

Today, we have all the world's knowledge at our fingertips—from the magic rectangle we carry around. But separating facts from fiction can be difficult.

Libraries actually have an amazing high-tech feature the Internet doesn't yet have. They keep all the nonfiction in one place, separate from the opinions and stories people make up. All with simple labels so you can tell what's true and what isn't. I'm still waiting for that from the Internet.

Books have an amazing way of sorting information that goes deeper into a subject than a ten-minute video can. But to be fair, YouTube is slowly becoming the new public lecture hall and Wikipedia the new open textbook.

Many dream of making the perfect educational system that will solve every student's problems. Unfortunately, every bad experience people have in school can be traced back to a well-intentioned person who thought they were making the perfect system. If you or someone you know has learning challenges, I suggest cultivating a passion for self-directed learning. There will never be a one-size-fits-all system that can hold a candle to freedom and passion combined.

The first thing I read at the library was not science or history or litera-ture. That's not how curiosity works. I went to the comic aisle and picked up Frank Miller's *Batman: Year One*—one of the greatest comics of all time. It showed a gritty, realistic view of Batman using skills and techniques to defeat others. Batman also was one of the first fictional brainhackers, learning every mental technique he could to get an edge.

Near the beginning of the book, right after Bruce Wayne's parents were murdered, Alfred was talking to another adult about him. Bruce can be seen in the background reading a book. I remember it reminded me of how adults would talk about me, right in front of me as if I wasn't there. The panel zoomed in to show the title of the book he was reading—*The Art of Lipreading*. His eyes were focused on the adults, not the book. This was a subtle way of saying that he knew everything people said about him, and he was still following his own path.

I had hearing problems from some of my past health issues. Surgeries did nothing, and I struggled to understand people through background noise. So, this made me think, *Could I really learn to lip-read?* Turns out, there were books on the subject right there in the library. I quickly did my best gritty Bruce Wayne impression and opened one up.

I didn't realize the extent of my hearing issues until I started to lip-read and caught the words that I was missing. Later, I would spend hours prac-ticing, looking at others and piecing together their conversations.

LIPREADING MADE EASY

Lipreading is the art of decoding the shape of mouths while combining this information with sporadic sounds to create a full picture of what a person is saying. The technique comes from the idea that the human mouth can only create a limited number of sounds, and there is a corresponding shape to each sound. For the purposes of lipreading, English only uses ten basic consonant types, and a limited number of vowels.

When asked what a vowel is, most people can't provide a proper answer beyond "A, E, I, O, U, and sometimes Y." A vowel is any sound that doesn't get interrupted by the tongue, teeth, or lips. It flows through. According to this definition, *w*, *h*, and *y* are actually vowels—not just sometimes.

You may think that ten consonants are not enough sounds. There are twenty-six letters in the alphabet, after all. That is where variations come in. Many sounds cover more than one letter. For example, the letters P and B represent variations of the same basic sound, as do T and D—one has a harder sound than the other. These pairs produce the same mouth shape too. The letters J, SH, and CH represent different sounds but all have nearly the same basic mouth position as well.

Each sound corresponds to a mouth shape formed by the relation between the tongue, teeth, and lips. By recognizing these mouth shapes, you can grasp most speech. It's not perfect, though. When reading lips, it's impossible to tell the letter variations apart, so the words *dial* and *tile* look the same. That's why context matters, and those little sounds caught here and there help.

To add one more challenge, some of the ten basic consonant types look the same (e.g., *t* and *sh*), as the only thing that changes is the tongue position, and you can't see that by looking. I have missed it many times and called a Terry, Sherry. Mumbling and facial hair are also challenges, and my biggest pet peeve is when people try to talk to me while facing away or cover their mouth while eating, thinking they are rude. It's like hitting mute in the middle of a conversation for me.

Decode Mouth Shapes

Learn the following basic sounds.

Vowels: *a, e, i, o, u, w, h, y*

1. *t, d*
2. *n*
3. *m*
4. *r*
5. *l*
6. *sh, ch, j, soft g*
7. *k, q*
8. *v, f*
9. *b, p*
10. *s, z*

Step One—Recognize: Open up your field of view and take in the entire face while looking for mouth shapes. Notice, for example, how even the jaw opens a bit for the L sound.

Step Two—Look for Context: As sounds start to become words for you, remember that you can be fooled. You will swear that they said a word when it was a trick of the mind. Many words look alike, so you will need context to understand.

Step Three—Practice: Turn down the volume on a sitcom, news, soap, or any programming where they show the whole face. Watch people's lips and try to piece together what they say.

One day it will just click.

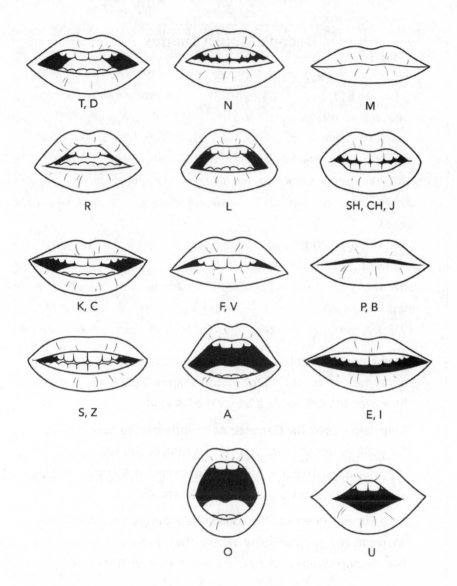

For these reasons, it's very hard to read lips with no vocal input at all. But beyond a few misunderstandings and with a few helpful echoes, you can comfortably follow a conversation across a crowded room if you want. It can be amazing.

Lipreading is second nature now for me. In fact, I only realize I'm doing it when a person points out that I am focusing on their lips. Crowded places like the bus completely changed from a place so noisy I had no idea what was going on to a joy. Everyone was facing the same direction with just the right amount of background echoes that I could now decode, allowing me to follow just about any conversation from the front of the bus. I was doing this for fun and practice, but stopped after I overheard/saw a surprising conversation between two old ladies that would make a sailor blush.

If you think this chapter does not apply to you, then give it time. We will all have to overcome physical challenges at some point. People in the disabled community refer to so-called able-bodied people as "temporarily able-bodied" because time and age come for us all. Except for me; I plan to live forever.

I also believe everyone has a challenge in their lives. We give up before trying, thinking there is no solution. If you have a challenge you want to overcome, take a moment and decide to look for answers. Some may be in this book, and others are beyond. My goal is to give you powerful brain-hacks and the roadmap to make your own solutions beyond what I teach. And if you develop a bit more compassion for others struggling with a challenge, then that's a good thing.

CHAPTER **SUMMARY**

- By learning mouth shapes, we can decode speech with our eyes and know what others are saying. It helps to have a few sounds and context though.

27 | Lie Detector

My Guinness Record was printed in the 1996 edition, and I was riding high emotionally. I had decided to turn this memory skill into a business but had absolutely no idea how to do that.

I thought the Guinness Record would change everything, I imagined the sky opening up and dropping money down. How could I be so smart and dumb at the same time? Looking back, I should have looked for a mentor or guide in business, but I experienced so much anger and animosity about the very idea of being self-employed, and I had to fight so hard to be taken seriously, that I didn't take the time to strategize.

So, after breaking the record, I took a year off to figure things out, pay the bills, and basically get into a rut. I got a basic service job making food. I made wraps for drunk people after the bars closed. It was actually a lot of fun, and I loved the people I worked with. Until one day, they accused me of stealing.

I entered work early one day to see the bosses (husband and wife) sitting down talking. They had counted the till and were just about to leave; so was Yolanda, the lady who worked the afternoon shift before me. I made myself comfortable, sitting next to the wall to wait when, almost by chance, I looked over to the till and saw Yolanda pulling a $20 bill out of the register. In plain sight. Not even trying to hide it. She was calm and smiled right at me as her eyebrows raised and lowered quickly, just after she saw me.

For a moment, I thought she was stealing, but her confidence made me feel like I was wrong. Maybe she had just made a change for a bigger bill or was told to take cab fare out of the till?

Without touching the register, I asked the bosses if they counted the till before my shift. They said they did, and everything was okay, so I dropped my suspicious mind and went to the bathroom to change. I did the shift without problems and the next day was told I was fired.

My request to have them count the till had backfired. Instead of clearing my mind of suspicion, it made them think I was covering up something. When I went to change, they had counted the register again. By this time, Yolanda was gone and by counting again, they discovered the till was missing that $20. I was accused of stealing even though I hadn't touched the till the entire time.

It sucks when your filler job that you don't like rejects you. I was only there while I figured out my business plan. It felt strange. I was so mad and humiliated. I was the best in the world at memory training. My program was unlike any other. I had literally invented new techniques and revolutionized the art of memory, and I was fired from a minimum wage job for stealing twenty bucks.

It was, of course, the best thing to ever happen to me. Without that job to fall back on, I was forced out of my comfort zone, and threw myself into making my business work. If I hadn't done that, I don't know where I would be today.

MICROEXPRESSIONS

Years later, I was hanging out with friends from McGill University's neuroscience department. They told me about tiny movements people make after they lie. Like a subconscious acknowledgment that they got caught. I remembered that little movement Yolanda's eyebrows made when I caught her taking the money out of the till. It was a microexpression.

As the story was told to me, scientists were trying to find out if some people could be natural lie detectors. So, they set up an experiment first by getting people to lie. They took two cups of liquid, one with sugar water and the other with vinegar in it. But both liquids were dyed to have exactly the same red color. While being filmed, each subject would drink from a random cup and either lie or tell the truth about the taste. Then, after the researchers had their footage, they showed it to people from all walks of life. It seemed that no one was the magical lie detector that they were looking for—until they tested some people in law enforcement. Some were FBI; others were border guards, but the result was the same. They were able to detect the liars with alarming accuracy. Sometimes perfect scores.

Lie Detector Hack

Step One: Observe the person without looking away. Microexpressions are usually in the face, but they can also involve a body movement, like a foot moving.

Step Two: Look for a movement that occurs one beat after they finish talking. Almost like they want you to believe them, so their body is asking a question a second after speaking.

Step Three: After the movement happens, the individual returns to their normal behavior, so filter out movements that are larger or longer-running, like standing up to get a drink of water. Microexpressions move, and then stop fast.

Step Four: Practice. This is a subtle art, so don't jump to a conclusion the first time you do this. We can see what we want to see and also misinterpret nervousness as dishonesty.

The results were so strong that researchers stopped the study to directly ask these super lie detectors how they became so good at this. Many talked about poker.

In poker, when a person gives away that they're lying, they have a "tell." This is usually a slight movement they make that gives away that they are being deceptive. No one gets lied to more often than law enforcement, and as a result of this daily practice at searching for tells, they became extremely good at pinpointing these microexpressions. They taught the scientists what to look for.

SOME VERBAL CUES OF DISHONESTY

Microexpressions are a visual cue that a person may be telling a lie. There are verbal cues to predict lying, but they should be taken with a grain of salt. It's like when the weatherman says there is a 50% chance of rain. You just want to know if you need an umbrella, but that's not how probabilities work.

The following cues are not just anecdotal, but were discovered by rigorous computer analysis of thousands of transcripts involving known lies and known truths. When people lie, they use distinct speech patterns, because the brain works differently when constructing a lie than when it's recalling the truth.

Disclaimer: The Lie Detector Hacks described are used by trained professionals and presented here for educational purposes. Occasionally, people who tell the truth will display some of these lying behaviors, and vice versa. Use these at your own risk.

Avoiding Personal Pronouns

When a person lies, they try to distance themselves from the story to avoid blame. So, they avoid using the word "I" or any self-reference and are less likely to call others by their names as well. This is believed to be part of the guilt mechanism. For example, if you heard a child lie about breaking a window they would talk about "those kids over there were goofing around and started throwing things. Then the one guy broke the window." If he were telling the truth, it would sound like, "I didn't break the window. I wasn't even there."

Giving Proof of Their Virtue

Normally, logic is not a bad thing, but liars are trying to push away blame and will try to tell you *why* they should be trusted. They will bring up unrelated topics and actions to construct an image of them as a trustworthy person. This is part of the desire to distance themselves from the event too. Sometimes I wonder if this means the modern act of virtue-signaling hides an inner hypocrisy in people.

Negative Language

A common tactic of liars is to avoid blame by blaming something else. Instead of just saying they are late because they slept in, it's the alarm clock's fault and the traffic, etc. If you hear someone try too hard to complain about things surrounding the event, they could be avoiding the spotlight themselves. This is partially an attempt to excuse the behavior too. There would be more examples of lying behavior here, but this darn computer just keeps acting up, the battery sucks, and . . .

* * *

One day, a couple of years after I was fired for Yolanda's theft, I saw her again. I was going to the bank to deposit some cash from my latest memory and speed-reading event. I was doing seminars for bigger crowds each time, and I had built up to a stack of thousands of dollars. As I walked to the bank, I resisted the urge to make it rain.

But I nearly dropped the envelope when I was in line. The next teller was Yolanda! I had so many mixed emotions. I wondered how the hell she was trusted to handle money. I was angry at her still, but thankful too, because I would not have this new life as an entrepreneur without her stealing. Her dishonesty led me to leave the safety of a job and go out on my own with great success. It kicked me out of the rut I was in then.

Ultimately, I settled on being grateful. This moment made me realize how much my life had changed for the better, and all because of her. As I got to the front of the line, she waved me over to the next teller. I invited the lady behind me to go instead of me and waited for the next teller. I may be grateful, but I'm not stupid.

CHAPTER **SUMMARY**

- The most common way to tell if someone is lying is to look for a small expression or movement they make a second after the lie.
- In data analyses of transcripts comparing lies and truth, some trends appeared, including avoiding personal pronouns, attempting to prove virtue, and using negative language.

AXIOM TWELVE
MIND OVER BODY

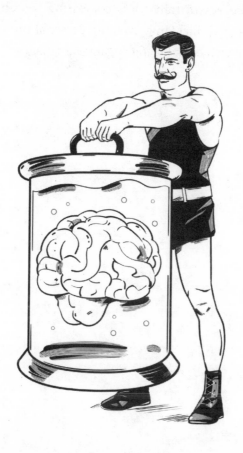

The body responds to our thoughts on a deeper level than one might think. The mind-body connection allows you to take control of physical processes. Everything from an immune response to bending steel has a power-up starting in the mind.

28 | Hack Cravings

Driving to and from the office, I would see it every day. Its siren song constantly compelling me to stop and order one. I tried to ignore it, but the sweet goodness was sitting there at the last turn before the highway. And I couldn't resist the chocolatey goodness.

Wendy's Frosty.

By about 2016, my business, Farrow Communications, had grown to cover brain training and marketing services, filling an office in Buffalo, New York. Like many in their late thirties, I had settled into a regular commute. Farrow Communications had grown into a well-respected PR and marketing firm, but my waistline grew along with it.

They say the metabolism slows down at this age, and there is nothing I can do about it. Problem is, I've heard people say things like that about everything else in my life and be wrong, so I wasn't ready to surrender to "dad bod."

It started with cravings, which start in the brain. I would discover that where the mind goes, the body follows. Almost every night when I drove home, I would have a Wendy's Frosty, piling on the pounds while congratulating myself for resisting this sweet treat on the way to the office that morning. The sheer joy of this drug hitting my brain rippled pleasure and erased the stress of the day. Or so I thought. One day, I stepped on the scale. I am a big guy—195 pounds when I graduated high school. Through weight training, I had been able to maintain that weight, and I had a lot of muscle, so I never thought I could become fat. But when I stepped on the scale, the dial must have been a *Star Trek* fan because it traveled where it had never gone before—past 200, past 220, boldly going all the way to 260. I went from muscular to chubby to larger than I was comfortable with; I had gained over sixty pounds in under eight months.

It was a tough year. My stress was high. We'd just had a baby, and I was running two businesses. In addition, we had a neighbor who was taking it as his personal mission to file complaints with the city over the height of our lawn instead of just talking to us directly like an adult. (Later, I would find out they wanted to buy the house we had just purchased.) Anyway, the stress and commute had played havoc on my chronic pain, especially my back pain, causing spasms and sleeplessness. This is what stopped me from exercising, causing more weight gain, which caused more pain in a negative cycle. I have pain in my knees and generally low energy during the day, but I was lucky to get four hours of sleep a night.

So, I deserved the treat, didn't I? The Frosty and other junk foods were my escape! And as my gut grew, I justified it. *My dad had a bigger gut at this age. It's natural.* But I knew in my heart that this wasn't true. I believe life is to be lived on purpose, despite what may happen to you. And life will knock you down. You will get good breaks and bad ones. Ultimately, the only thing you have control over is yourself, and what you do, more than anything else, determines the course of your life. So, when it comes to what I put in my mouth, I'm in control, right? Not exactly.

The problem with being smart is that you know when you're lying to yourself. I could see the cycles, and I had a choice.

VIRTUOUS VS. DESTRUCTIVE CYCLES

"The means may be likened to a seed, the end to a tree; and there is just the same inviolable connection between the means and the end as there is between the seed and the tree."
—Mahatma Gandhi, *Indian Home Rule*

Believing in change does not mean being ignorant of how life works. We are products of causation. One event causes another, and our life clicks forward like dominos. That's why it helps to see things we want to change as cycles rather than traits.

Negative cycles happen more often because it's easier to destroy progress than it is to build it up. One time falling off the wagon or skipping leg day can lead to more negative results. The longer this goes on, the harder it is to break the cycle.

The first step was to get rid of my craving for a Frosty.

There was one brainhack I hadn't tried yet—a hack that works so well, I'd avoided it because I knew from experience that if I used this hack, I would never eat a Frosty again. And I was right.

It's the Disgust Hack.

The Disgust Hack

Trick your brain into hating specific foods.

Warning: This trick isn't for the faint of heart. You will imagine disgusting things and transfer that feeling to the food. The downside is that it ruins that food for you. This isn't a subtle trick. There is no way to do this by halves. It's all or nothing. In my experience, if you do it right, you should lose all desire for that food forever.

Step One: Imagine the food you like in all its forms. Make a mental film of every step of making and eating the food, from the first smell to tossing the wrapper away.

Step Two: Add a list of disgusting things to the food as you mentally eat it. Try motor oil, vomit, and more. What really works for me is bugs or maggots. (I did say this technique isn't for the faint of heart.)

Step Three: Go through this visualization daily or even twice a day for at least a month.

Step Four: Make peace with the loss. You will *not* like that food anymore.

The Disgust Technique is good for a specific food you are addicted to, and it will cancel one food from your palette at a time. It breaks the addiction. For instance, I stopped craving Wendy's Frostys right away. Even years later, after I forgot the imagery I created, my desire for that item is still gone. As a test, I tried a Frosty just before writing this chapter, and I couldn't finish it. That is the power of the brain. But the trick doesn't transfer—I still eat ice cream.

* * *

This brainhack was helpful, and I felt empowered, but it was just the first step to getting healthy again. If I did nothing, similar foods would take the place of the Frosty, so doing this for an entire diet is like a mental game of whack-a-mole. Plus, I wanted to enjoy some junk food in moderation and really just needed the cravings to stop.

THE BELLY BRAIN

Over the last few years, research on weight loss has changed dramatically. We now understand the role DNA plays in the process as well as the human microbiome and the role of the brain in your belly.

The brain is the governor of the body. So, if weight loss is to be effective, it starts in the brain.

Diets don't work because of the brain's governing mechanism. No matter the diet, they all involve some kind of food restriction without any consideration of the brain and body's reaction to being restricted. Temporarily restricting foods causes little change, but after a point is reached where your brain thinks is enough, then the brain counters the restriction to go back to its ideal state. This breaks the diet. There are a few notable exceptions to this, like when someone makes a diet change into a form of identity (like being vegetarian or following religious dietary rules).

There are also occasions where people get medical news that scare them into changing their habits. When my dad was diagnosed with chronic obstructive pulmonary disease, he instantly had to stop smoking, and he also started dieting. He was able to do it successfully and kept the weight off because it was life or death to him. I am forever grateful that he did.

So, to lose weight, I had to get my brain to change first.

After that, the body will follow.

Taste Hack

The next brainhack I wanted to try related to how the body senses food. We know the brain doesn't have an objective measure for hot versus cold, fast versus slow, or sweet versus bland (as you'll recall from the speed-reading chapters). Instead, these subjective values come from comparing what we're eating now to the general diet we have been eating for the last few months.

Think of any time you were told that a food was an acquired taste. Just look at YouTube videos on people eating *salmiakki* (super salty licorice) or very spicy foods. Eating these things results in slow changes to tastebuds over time—in some cases, getting used to a flavor that would make others vomit.

The point is, we get used to flavors over time, not all at once. Interestingly, oftentimes people who like spicy and bitter flavors are leaner than those who like sweets. That makes sense, of course—if you eat less sugar, you won't gain weight—but it's deeper than that.

If you cut back on sugar and sweet foods in general, you become more sensitive to the taste of sweet things. So, the irony is that if you eat a lot of sugar, you don't really enjoy it as much as a person who eats a little. Your taste buds become desensitized, requiring more and more to get the same sweet feeling. So, instead of dieting, I focused on making my taste for sugar more sensitive. I started adding bitter foods to my diet (like cooking with vinegar and lemon juice) and cut back on added sugar by having my daily coffee black. There was an adjustment period, but soon I was enjoying it, and noticed that sweet foods tasted much sweeter than they did in the past.

The same thing happens when you eat bland food for a long time, like during a hospital stay. The first steak you eat will feel like there are fireworks going off in the background.

This is not a diet. It's a step-by-step way to change how taste works. You are slowly changing your brain.

Another fun thing you can do with this principle is to confuse the senses by alternating flavors. My favorite combination was sweet and spicy. Having something spicy between bites of sweet things meant only a tiny bit of sweetness tasted like it was packed with sugar. My favorite was a sweet and spicy salmon recipe.

CHAPTER **SUMMARY**

- End a food addiction by imagining eating that food with something that disgusts you. The two things get linked, and you never feel the same about it.
- The sense of taste can be hacked by doing things like lowering sweeteners and swapping flavors.

29 | Don't Follow Your Gut. Lead It.

A poem for a microbiome:
Cut sugar and carbs for a week,
The cravings can become meek,
But fast over a day, and it falls away.
It's a brainhack, not a sundae, you seek.

Every time I dropped below a certain weight—my set point weight, which I'll explain in a moment—I felt physically better. My pain was lower, and I had more energy. But I had terrible cravings. They didn't correspond to anything I was doing. I got them at all weight levels. When the cravings kicked in, I would eat to the point of pain. It seemed like I couldn't stop eating, even when I was full.

I was like the guy in the Monty Python movie *The Meaning of Life*. He kept eating till he was full, then the waiter gave him a wafer-thin mint. It was just enough to make him explode. I felt like that regularly.

I would discover that it was my microbiome that was to blame, but the solution was still in the brain. This is usually where a diet plan says it's not your fault, and you are powerless to your cravings. In a sense, that's true. But even though it isn't your fault, that does not mean you are powerless to change it.

Note: Consult a doctor before trying anything you read in this book. I am only recounting what worked for me.

SET POINT

Research on weight loss has discovered that everyone seems to have a "set point"—the weight that their body feels most comfortable at. People diet and lose weight but often return to this point. However, most of this research doesn't account for the brain and other sources of the set point, like the human microbiome. I have found that the set point can actually be changed, and like other subconscious bodily functions, the solution is found partially in the brain but also in the microbiome. More on that later.

So, I was using brainhacks to cut back on sugar and was able to lower my "set point" weight back to my original 200 pounds. The set point is a magic number that diet researchers see as the body's "thermostat" for weight. By changing taste sensitivity and using other brainhacks, I could move my set point over time. But there was another factor happening beyond that. I would eat well for a while then get those incredible cravings again. This was not about losing weight anymore; it was about feeling better. I joked about how it was beyond my brain—like someone else was controlling me. I was right. It was my microbiome.

I learned about this from my wife Andrea. She was an amazing role model for weight loss. After having our first child, she gained weight, and then lost it, and then lost some more while gaining muscle. Right now, she is under 100 pounds (yes, really) and is fitter and healthier than she was before she lost the weight, and many health problems she dealt with before—from migraines to backaches—disappeared after her weight loss. She even challenges me to chin-up competitions on a regular basis. Of course, 100 pounds isn't a healthy goal for every single person, but science tells us the less fat you have, the longer you live. This is true in my wife's family: her granny maintains a healthy weight and is still gardening and living on her own at 88. There is a saying that you don't see overweight people in their nineties for a reason.

The first thing I learned from Andrea is to not feel guilt or shame or any feelings about your body. Just see it like a machine. Andrea didn't exercise or follow a formal diet. She trained her brain to focus on portion sizes and also occasionally fasted. She never ate a meal bigger than the size of her fist. She hoped that over time she would shrink her stomach and not need as much food. It worked. Portion control is not about what you eat, it's about developing your eating habits via brain training. The small portions and fasting also killed off harmful bacteria in her stomach biome, getting rid of bad cravings. She posted about her results to Facebook, and many started to copy her plan with success. But most of the feedback was negative. She taught me about the double standard women experience in the crab bucket. When a guy does three push-ups, he gets high fives and respect from male friends. But when she talked about fasting and portion control, people responded with judgment and even anger, as if she was hurting other women by showing pictures of her results. She calls it "skinny shaming." I will never understand the stupidity of the crab bucket as long as I live.

Portion control worked for her and many others, so I experimented with it, but it didn't work for me. Every time I ate a little bit, the cravings would kick in and make me crave more. But she was doing something else. She was changing her microbiome. By fasting from time to time and eating biome-helping foods like garlic, she got rid of bacteria in her gut that were causing cravings. It turns out the cravings we often feel for sugar are not coming from our brains. They come from the little creatures in our guts. A specific set of microbiome creatures eat sugar and then excrete a hormone that makes you hold onto fat and crave sugar. When you eat sugar, they multiply and make you crave more in a destructive cycle. The reason for my crazy cravings was a bug inside me telling me to crave it. Time for a brainhack to take back control.

You may have noticed by now that most of the cool superhuman-like tools in this book have their roots in understanding our primitive history. We have the same brain and body (for the most part) that cavemen and women did while hunting mammoths. The difference between then and now is that food was not available all the time back then. For most of human history, food came in cycles of feast and famine. Living off a few seeds for a week waiting for berries to ripen or for a kill from a hunt was common. In essence, living back then was a form of intermittent fasting. The cells attuned to this cycle too. During the feast time, the cells store as many calories as possible, but during the famine, they switch to repair the cells and DNA. This division of time and effort still goes on in your cells to this day.

Data shows that groups of people who undergo short periods of starvation experience tremendous health benefits—from improving the symptoms of many ailments to even lowering your biological age. I want to make a distinction between this and actual starvation. There are many people who don't have access to the nutrition they need, and that is terrible. However, here, I'm talking about a natural cycle that was fueled by the changing of the seasons.

Fasting Brainhacks

So, you want to fast. But unfortunately, no diet book focuses on the real thing that is controlling your eating: your brain. Here are some brainhacks to make it easier.

Cold Turkey Timer

Of all the methods to stop smoking or drinking, research suggests that the hack that works most often is simply quitting cold turkey. Having one rule makes it easier for your brain to follow, and due to brain plasticity, after a period of adjustment, the body will get used to it. The problem, of course, is that you can't quit food cold turkey, but intermittent fasting is the next best thing. Set a time of day that you will eat and a time you will stop. Adjust this over time.

For example, I started by just eliminating my midnight snacks. I stopped eating at 9 p.m. and didn't start until 9 a.m. the next day.

Then I moved 9 a.m. to noon, and then to 2 p.m., with the help of the next hack.

Fill Your Stomach

The easiest way to stick to a fasting schedule is to get into the habit of drinking a lot of fluid early in the day. This is great for our bodies, because we wake up dehydrated and coffee only makes it worse. I drink a bottle of tea every morning. No sugar. It helps me feel full until at least noon. Even with a full belly, there will be tough times that hunger calls. So, push it away.

Push Away Hunger

Remember the Push Away Pain Brainhack from the beginning of the book? Well, you can use it to push away hunger too. Visualize the area and imagine what the hunger looks like and breathe deeply while you push it away from you. This will help for the tough times. Stick to this long enough for the brain to change.

Plasticity Brainhack

Just about everyone who tries fasting says they get used to it over time. That is brain plasticity at work. I often say willpower is for losers (because you will lose). Real change comes from changing your brain over time. In other words, willpower does not work because the body fights back. But focusing on developing the habit of fasting is easier to get used to.

The Sugar Fast

Though not technically a brainhack, this is a strategy I used in the beginning, so I'm including it here. At first, I could not fast for long periods of time at all. I would do well for a while, and then the cravings would kick in. Knowing the cravings came from bacteria whose numbers were boosted by sugar made me try the next best thing. I couldn't starve myself, but I could maybe starve them a bit to gain back control. So, I cut out sugar of all kinds for a week. It's important to note that sugar in this context also includes nearly all carbs from bread to potatoes, because they are converted into sugars in the body. I tried this for a week: strictly eating no more than twenty grams of carbs or sugar a day. I actually ate a lot that week—mostly high-protein snacks but almost no carbs. Then, I ate normally for a month, and the results were incredible. The intense cravings I had were much less. I lost weight around my waist too. Then I was able to fast and lose even more.

The first step when planning to do this is to check in with your doctor and look at your lifestyle. Then, take time to choose the best fasting times for you and experiment to find the solution for you. Today, I'm fit and healthy—and I even overcame my chronic pain with a combination of stretching, exercise, and keeping my body fat low.

I think back to some friends I made in the Tibetan Buddhist community. They regularly fasted, and their energy and vitality were legendary well into their seventies and beyond. The fasting seems to have a large impact on the microbiome too. After fasting, the harmful bacteria start to die off, creating a better bacterial balance in the gut.

I was sure this bacteria was the cause of my problem. I had "sugar-addicted bacteria."

Luckily, they *can* be killed, and this brainhack helps it happen.

I still eat sweets from time to time, but I don't get the cravings I used to get. I don't eat when full or till my stomach hurts, and most importantly, if I do gain weight, over the holidays for example, I can lose it just as quickly and easily now. That's the key for me. It's not about having a perfect body, it's about actually being in control of my body.

I hope this chapter gives others hope to keep looking for answers to their challenges and not to give up. It's easy to give up or blame others, society, genetics, and even your gut. I hope my readers are braver than that. After all, brainhacks are just tools in your toolbox. You are the builder that uses them.

CHAPTER **SUMMARY**

- The most effective method to quit a bad habit is cold turkey. There is a period of adjustment, but then the body adapts.
- Like the Push Away Pain Brainhack from earlier, you can push away hunger to stick to your fast. Just follow the same steps.
- There are several hacks for controlling your eating. Instead of dieting, follow these.

30 | Strong-Body Brainhacks

J ust the other day, I found Lex in my workout area, a small addition on the back of the house where I added a few fun pieces of exercise equipment—monkey bars, gymnastic rings, a punching bag, and a Wing Chun dummy, to name a few. We call it the dojo. I was getting in better and better shape now that I had gotten used to fasting. So, I took up these exercises to build muscle, and it was working.

I was on the gymnastic rings when I saw Lex out of the corner of my eye trying to lift a plate that weighed 25 pounds. He was only seven, and weighed just 50 pounds himself. He tried once, then I tried to step in so he wouldn't hurt himself. "Hey son, I have an idea."

"No, Dad, I got this," he said, talking like a YouTuber he likes.

He tried a second time, and it moved a tiny bit . . . like Captain America pulling on Thor's hammer in *Avengers: Age of Ultron*.

"I have a suggestion."

"I want to try one more time," Lex gasped as he adjusted his grip. His next attempt was a quick pull that made the weight jump up just before he lost his balance and fell forward. Huffing and sighing like a man in his forties, he turned to me. "Okay, Dad. What's the brainhack for this?"

I smiled. "What makes you think there's a brainhack for lifting weights, son?"

"Because you always have a brainhack when you talk like that." He was brooding now, upset he hadn't figured it out himself.

Meanwhile, I was doing exactly what I disliked about others when I was a kid. I was talking down to him. I quickly decided that it was time to change tack.

"Would it make you feel better if I told you I only learned this after years of trying it the wrong way?"

"A little," Lex said.

"What if I told you this brainhack was developed in circuses and used by the Russians during the Cold War?"

"Like Black Widow!" he exclaimed. Marvel references seem to be more common than water these days, so I went with it.

I walked over to the back of the dojo where I kept some workshop material, and grabbed a piece of rebar, the kind of steel used in the foundation of buildings to reinforce concrete. At the same time, I handed him a smaller, aluminum bar. It was softer and smaller, but it still would be a challenge for him.

"Years ago, circuses used to have strongmen. They would lift heavy items and perform feats of strength that were amazing for the time. This is a brainhack that they used. They would bend steel bars and nails with their hands. They would challenge body builders to do the same thing, and they couldn't do it because they didn't know the brainhack."

"How can a brainhack make you have bigger muscles?" Lex asked.

"Not bigger muscles—this brainhack makes all your muscles fire together and brings out more strength."

I told Lex to hold the aluminum bar against his hip because the right angle was key. If I held the bar in front of me and just tried to bend it with my hands, it wouldn't budge because my hands aren't strong enough. I made a grunting sound as I held the bar out in front of me like Superman making a power pose and attempted to bend it. It's impossible. He copied me to confirm I was telling the truth. *Good*, I thought. I like it when he is skeptical and wants to confirm things himself. It means he's teaching himself, not just listening to a lecture.

ELECTRIC MUSCLES

First, we each tried to bend the bar against our hip. It flexed, but did not bend. I told him that there was a brainhack to unlock more power. It's a neurological trick.

Our muscles are powered by electricity, but they are actually much stronger than we think. The brain holds back most of this strength because it wants to be efficient. This is why we sometimes hear stories of moms rolling cars off their kids: because, in that moment of extreme emergency, the brain takes off all the safety blocks and gives the muscles full power.

"How can we get the power of a mom, then?" Lex asked, and it made me laugh. He laughed along, understanding what he'd said. "I mean that mom who lifted the car," he corrected. "How do we get that power?"

"By tensing our whole body in pulses," I replied, knowing I would have to explain more. "This is when you tense your muscles all at once. That means every muscle in your body from head to toe. This activates more energy and channels more electricity into the muscles you want to use."

The interesting thing is that, unlike powering electric motors, you don't lose power by activating more muscles. Instead, your body actually gives you more energy. So, tense all your muscles as you work to bend the metal, and you will be stronger. Lifting weights while tensing your abs and back are also good for your body and prevent injury.

Muscle-Mind Hack

Our muscles hold back most of our power to be efficient and avoid injury. Simply tense all the surrounding muscles during a lift, and the muscle doing the work gets more electricity. This tricks the brain into sending out more energy. If you tense the whole body, you can get a bigger boost, but be careful and don't hurt yourself.

Lex tried this, and bent the bar a tiny bit. It was time for the final technique to bring this lesson home.

PULSES

"Now the pulse contractions," I said. "When circus strongmen would lift heavy items and perform amazing feats of strength, they used this trick. After offering audience members the chance to bend a bar with no luck, they would take it back, put it against their hips, and do the full-body contractions just like I taught you. But in pulses."

Pulses Brainhack

Instead of applying steady pressure against a bar, tense and relax every muscle in a second, and then repeat this over and over to trick your body into generating and concentrating power during that one moment.

The idea is that by pulsing, the brain activates more muscle fibers and makes you stronger. Another theory about why it works is that force equals mass times acceleration. So, trying to attack the end of the bar faster creates more initial force. This helps overcome inertia.

By the end of my lecture, I held up a steel bar bent into a U shape. Looking down, I saw Lex hold up his own bar, bent fully, with a smile of pride on his face.

"Good job," I said with equal pride.

THE STRETCHING HACK

This next hack is more than a circus trick. It helped me overcome my chronic pain. A lot of pain comes from a lack of flexibility, and for me it was in my hamstrings. Our bodies react to every stress with tension, because in the wild, tension is nature's first aid.

Whether you break a bone, get stabbed, or just stub your toe, the automatic body response to injury is almost identical. You make a loud noise and hold the injured area as tensely as possible.

The noise alerts others that you need help while the tension stops blood flow and holds the area firmly in place to avoid further injury. This response is genius . . . unless you happen to create a civilization that constantly causes people stress without leaving leisure time to relax. This triggers more and more tension that pulls on our joints causing pain.

Whether you do yoga or traditional stretching, or special exercises designed by a physiotherapist, gentle stretching has benefits all over the body. But for most people, it seems impossible. If a person hasn't stretched for most of their life, it will be very painful.

This is where I found myself in my late thirties; my back pain led to more and more tension and pain in my body. Over the years, my hamstrings especially were being subjected to more and more tension, which was pulling on my back, causing more pain and damage. Combined with the inflammation I had, it was tough. Finally, a physiotherapist showed me that my body was getting less flexible over time. He sent me home to do a series of stretches. But when I tried to stretch, the pain was even sharper. It was excruciating. It felt like I was being stabbed in the leg. Stretching these muscles hurt, and that caused them to tense up and hurt even more the next day. Finally, after weeks of daily practice, I was tenser than when I'd started—and ready to give up. I had felt pain before, but this pain was so sharp and intense that I had to find another way.

Then, one night, I had a dream. I'm not kidding or exaggerating. I was in a yoga studio and not doing my stretching well. The instructor said, "Your brain tells your body what to do. Your brain governs the tension." Then I woke up and did some research. The solution to my challenge came from an old Cold War–era program in Russia. I discovered that the relationship between tension and relaxation in the body originates in the brain.

We often think of innovation as being a product of a free economy. But innovation is the product of a free *mind* solving a problem. In Communist Russia, resources were scarce. Redistributing everything seemed to get everyone less than they needed to survive, except the Communist Party officials, of course. For many poor people, sports were their way out of this horrible system. Getting to the international stage meant a stipend from the government, better housing, and other benefits. Athletes were given an incentive to metaphorically punch Rocky in the mouth.

This, of course, led to insane training methods and many drug scandals, but also genius innovation. The Russians took the ideas of pulsing and tension used by circus strongmen to a whole new level.

They didn't have the Americans' wealth of equipment, so they delved deeper into experimenting with training methods to achieve peak performance. This led to a breakthrough used today in gyms around the world. They discovered that tension is governed by a nervous system that tries to protect the muscles in the body. And it has a hack.

Stretching-Mind Hack

Every muscle in our body has a point to which it's comfortable stretching. If you put your leg up on a table and lean toward your toes, there will be a sudden point when tension prevents you from going farther. We know that the muscle itself can go much farther based on its length. So, it's the software that governs the leg, telling it to stop at that place. This point is chosen to protect your leg from injury, and it can change depending on your position.

Take a moment and compare how far you can reach—to your toes, the floor, etc.—while standing and bending over vs. how close you get with one leg elevated on a table or bar. Even though it's the exact same muscle involved, the elevated leg often lets you go much farther because bending in that direction has less risk of injury.

Tension is like the software of the brain and nervous system, not a function of the body. The software is called the governor. For example, it governs your leg, telling you how far you can stretch without stopping. Push any further, and it will just tense more to stop you. This tension is subconscious. You have no direct control over it. But there is a hack for it.

> The Russians discovered that when you willfully tense your muscles for ten seconds, the governor shuts off because tensing means it has no reason to activate. Then if you relax, there's a one-second window of time before the governor is turned back on. In that second, you can stretch much farther than normal, and if you hold the new position for thirty seconds, it trains the muscle to govern at that new level.
>
> Remember: Flexibility and tension are in the brain, not the body.

The other great part of this trick is that it helps a new stretcher make progress and train the body to relax. Many mind-body hacks take advantage of the space between your two nervous systems. The autonomic and voluntary systems. Voluntary is every time you move a muscle on purpose. You take control. Then, all the other functions like breathing and tension are governed by your subconscious autonomic system. That microsecond delay that the Russians discovered between when you tense and when the governor activates uses your voluntary system before your autonomic system kicks in.

I went back to my stretches using the tense and relax technique, and it worked. In just a week, I could get rid of the tension I had felt for years. After a month, I was almost doing the splits.

I now stretch every day, and it's changed my life. With just a technique, I removed the majority of chronic pain from my life.

CHAPTER **SUMMARY**

- With the Muscle-Mind Hack, simply tense all the surrounding muscles during a lift, and the muscle doing the work gets more electricity. This tricks the brain into sending out more energy. If you tense the whole body, you can get a bigger boost, but be careful and don't hurt yourself.

- Exerting muscles in pulses gives you strength you didn't know you had.
- Tension is held in the mind, not the body. People have tricked the mind into loosening up tension on a muscle by tensing for ten seconds then relaxing into a stretch. Some say they need a partner for this, but it's not necessary. Just be careful and consult your doctor to do it safely.

31 | Hacking Sleep

Start counting backward from 100," the nurse told me. *100, 99.* I feel the cold liquid fill the veins in my arm. *98, 97,* I start to drift off just as I become aware of my breathing. *96, 95.* I get scared at that moment, panicking because my body won't move. Then I wake up. I had another dream of the hospital. The clock reads 1:23 a.m. *Why can't I sleep? Why can't I sleep? What's wrong with me?* I thought. How can I suck at something I do every night? I'd had forty years of practice and couldn't get this right!?

I had been having insomnia ever since changing my sleep position. It was the last step to fixing my back pain. My natural position was face down with one leg up, but as I slept and my muscles relaxed, it twisted my back. I tried different sleep positions, and the only one that would work was side sleeping. It was perfect, my back felt great, and everything was supported. The only problem was that I couldn't seem to fall asleep in that position. I would lie awake in the perfect sleep position for hours without so much as a nap, but if I gave up and returned to my old position, I would have pain the next day. The choice was between insomnia or pain.

HYPER BRAIN

To be fair, I had insomnia for years on and off because of my hyper brain. It's a common problem for ADHD people, as well as those who are very mentally active or have a high IQ or overactive imaginations. As we drift off to sleep, the brain can flip into a state that becomes incredibly active, going over seemingly small matters with intense focus. The hyper brain concept was discovered by researchers to be a byproduct of an active imagination and mental activity during the day. Since the goal of this book is to teach you brainhacks to make you smarter, it makes sense to address one of the downsides of an active brain: the inability to turn it off.

Sleep Hygiene Brainhack

The first thing to do when facing insomnia is sleep hygiene. This covers everything that surrounds the act of sleeping. Turn off entertainment, avoid video games, and lower lights before sleep. Exercising a few hours before sleep can help too. Also, brainhackers should avoid doing focus bursts too close to sleep because that will trigger adrenalin that will stay in your system for hours.

Melatonin can be another simple part of sleep hygiene. It's a natural hormone released by the brain to trigger the sleep process. It is not a tranquilizer. But when we have artificial lights on like TVs and computers, our brain produces less of it. Consult a doctor before taking new supplements, but I decided to get the lowest dose of melatonin I could. You don't need much, and more does not make you fall asleep faster. It's only helpful to trigger sleep. If you take too much, it will stay in your system and make you drowsy the next day.

I got a few nights' sleep with these tips, but still felt uncomfortable, and it didn't help my hyper brain at all. The biggest problem is that hyper brain is not just junk-thinking or paranoia. The ideas you have while drifting off to sleep are often the best, most *important* ideas.

This is a natural phenomenon. In fact, everyone has experienced this feeling of brilliant ideas flooding them when their brain is otherwise inactive. Think of a time when you were in the shower, on a commute, or just drifting off to sleep. It seems that our mind waits for those quiet moments when the external world dies down to reveal the brilliant gem it's been saving for us all day. In one comic book, Tony Stark deals with hyper brain, and even Elon Musk talks about his struggles with it too.

Hyper Brain Journal Hack

Work and stress are a big part of hyper brain. During the day, we have so many things going on that when we finally relax and drift off, it gives our brain a chance to solve our problems. As it turned out, the best solution for me was a journal. I made a habit of writing down my thoughts at night and trying to get them all out before sleeping, and every morning, I would open up the book to go over the ideas. This trained my brain to let go of extra thoughts because they were safe and recorded, not just bouncing around in my head or pushing me to write an email. After journaling, I found myself ready to "shut down" as soon as my head hit the pillow. Just five to ten minutes of journaling was enough to work wonders.

BIPHASIC SLEEP

I was sleeping better, but still tired during the day, so I tried to split up my sleep. Since I had difficulty sleeping for eight hours all at once, I tried to break it up. Biphasic sleep is when you split your sleep cycles up into two different times throughout the day. So, instead of eight hours at night, you try four hours at night and four during the day. Sailors used this type of sleep schedule, training their brains to sleep for twenty minutes at a time so they could perform solo trips across the Atlantic. So, since I was already crashing in the afternoon, I thought I would try it. It takes about four days to get used to. However, it's natural for the brain, and anyone who has been an insomniac before is well-suited to this process.

It worked at first and felt fantastic. I would sleep until about 8 in the morning, then stay awake until about 4 in the afternoon, then sleep till 6 or 7. Then I could have a full evening and work right up until 4 a.m.

This biphasic sleep was working out great at first, because when I woke up at 6, I could spend time with my son and hang out with friends and family. I even had some leisure time until 9 or 10; then, I still had an entire shift of work after everyone had gone to bed. I'd get stuff accomplished, improve my business, and still be bright-eyed and bushy-tailed the next day at 8 a.m. when I had meetings to attend.

This was great. I felt on top of the world; I felt that I had conquered my sleep problem. It was wonderful . . . until date night happened.

In my infinite wisdom, I hadn't thought of what my wife wanted. For a date night, I tried to stay up through my second sleep time at 4 p.m. After that, my entire biphasic sleep schedule was destroyed. I just couldn't get back into the groove. It seems like biphasic sleep is a wonderful idea as long as you can be absolutely perfect with it. I couldn't.

If you have the right schedule—shift work, for instance—I highly recommend giving it a shot. It honestly feels like you have so much extra time in your life, and it's really cool to be awake when everyone else is asleep. Again, though, if you break your biphasic sleep cycle, it feels terrible.

I did settle into a nice afternoon nap of 30 minutes, which I still take to this day and which has amazing health benefits. There is a long list of famous brains that have taken regular afternoon naps, from Einstein to Ben Franklin. It really works.

LUCID DREAMS

I wanted to add a quick side note on lucid dreaming. Once you can sleep well, you should try to lucid dream. It's an amazing feeling that comes simply from being aware that you are dreaming. Once you wake up in your dream, you can do anything. My favorite activity is to fly around the sky.

Lucid dreaming is very unstable, and at first only lasts seconds, but over time you can hold it for longer. When you're in a lucid dream, anything you think of becomes reality. The easiest way to start lucid dreaming is to record your dreams. It's a technique that never fails to produce consistent lucid dreams. Keep a dream journal beside your bed, and when you wake up, start writing down your dreams. The first few times you try this, you may draw a blank, but keep trying. The next time, you may write a sentence . . . and then three the following morning. Soon, you'll be writing an entire page or more. I reached the point where I would recall up to six dreams a night, and I switched from writing to using a recording device because it was taking too much time to write it all out.

The content of the dream does not matter, and you will never need to read these dreams or listen to the recordings. It is the fact that the brain knows it will have to remember the dream that creates a change. At some point, you'll be in a dream and realize you need to remember this for later. Then your second thought will be instantly realizing that the world around you is made up.

Lucid dreams tend to be the last dream of the night, so don't use an alarm clock if you want to do this.

When you find yourself in the dream, the fact that you are awake in a dream will cause the world around you to become unstable. A little trick to make it stable again is to look at your hands. For whatever reason, looking at your hands will ground you. It brings you into the dream by convincing your brain that the dream is a real place. After that point, just keep practicing, and you can have lucid dreams that last a long time. Try flying in your dream as soon as you can. It's an amazing feeling.

HOW TO THINK OF NOTHING

After all of these steps, I still had nights that I could not shut my brain off. Then I realized that I never decided to shut it off. I still thought about my day, expecting sleep to overtake me. If you have difficulty sleeping, you know what I mean. It takes a conscious decision to stop thinking, but it's also a skill. You may not think it's possible to clear your mind, but it's actually a practice that's not difficult to master. Truth be told, I learned much of this from my friends in the Tibetan Buddhist community, whose meditation techniques are on another level. They were kind enough to welcome me to the temple to learn how they meditate and practice it myself.

There's an age-old saying that the one way to make sure that somebody thinks of a pink elephant is to tell them not to think of it. In other words, our brains tend to not have an "off" switch; instead, they jump from thought to thought. So, to slow the mind down, you need to tame it, so to speak.

Try this, for example: Think of a blank piece of paper. Just hold it in your mind for a second. It'll likely disappear or change a split second later because our minds are constantly active. When we try to visualize something, it tends to pop out of our heads as quickly as it pops in. This is normal. In meditation, monks will imagine an object like a lotus flower to tame their active minds.

Think of Nothing Hack

Step One: Decide to clear your mind. Write down any ideas you have or want to store to prepare yourself to stop thinking (i.e., journaling).

Step Two: Next, pick an object that you are familiar with that you can easily visualize—like a rock or a flower—and simply visualize it in your mind's eye. Your mind will change, twist it or bend it around . . . or replace it with any number of more important things your subconscious wants to tell you at that moment.

Step Three: Take a deep breath and try again. For the next few minutes, simply repeat this practice every time that image changes. Take a breath. Be mentally thankful for this information. Don't get irritated by it or see it as the enemy. Because it's not. Simply accept the distraction, and let it go as you breathe out and imagine your object again. As it says on the shampoo bottle, wash, rinse, repeat and repeat and repeat and repeat, and over time, you will notice that the image starts to stay. The image overpowers the distraction and there will be moments where you hold on to that image for a long time.

Step Four: Try keeping count without opening your eyes. Monks use beads to count their prayers. Many think the catholic rosary as the source of this practice but it's the other way around. Beaded and knotted rope dates back to early Tao and African religions using knotted ropes and beads to count prayers. In fact, the English word "bead" derives from an old word for prayer. But it's about more than counting prayers for penance. It trains the brain to focus by counting the number of times you lose the image you are trying to hold in your mind.

Step Five: Now, to clear your mind. The next step is to replace the blank page with a white background. That is, instead of imagining an object, imagine nothing—absolute empty space . . . no sound, no light. Nothingness. Don't focus on looking at the nothingness or being aware of the nothingness; let go of your focus and let your mind be free. Try this after you have made progress with the object meditation. Just like before, you're going to get distracted, and something will pop into your head. Not to worry, though. Taking a deep breath, let that unwanted thought drift out of your head, and go back to nothingness. With practice, you can maintain a mental state of nothingness for a long time. You will start to notice you forget trains of thought during this exercise. That is good. The goal is to get to the mindset of no thought. It feels absolutely amazing to reach.

This combined with counting backward solved my sleep problems. The counting backward gave me something to focus on, making it a lot easier to push away distractions than I would in a pure meditative state. I counted backward from one hundred, and when I got to one, I would start back at one hundred. I'd just simply count and clear my mind. Nothing existed in my mind except for the numbers. I noticed I was starting to fall asleep when I would make mistakes with my count, forgetting where I was. I didn't get upset because letting go is the point. Be happy that you lost track and let go completely. So far, it's only taken me two rounds of counting. By my second countdown, I was always asleep before I got to one.

CHAPTER **SUMMARY**

- One of the downsides of an active brain is the inability to turn it off—leading to sleeping issues.
- Sleep hygiene, such as turning off screens, exercising before bed, and taking a melatonin supplement, can help trigger sleep.
- Another hack is to get everything that's on your mind on paper before going to sleep. This trains the brain to let go of thoughts.
- Biphasic sleep means splitting up your sleep into two different times throughout the day. This is helpful especially for shift work.
- Just for fun, try writing down your dreams!
- The Think of Nothing Hack helps tame your brain to let go of thoughts.

AXIOM THIRTEEN

THE FARROW BRAIN MODEL

I believe that our brain is ruled by two forces. The function that creates connections and the one that compares them: the memory and the mirror. These two fates make the core of our identity, backed by chemical rewards and punishments. Though just a theory, this way of seeing the brain has led me to solid explanations for things like emotions, self-esteem, drive, luck, self-sabotage, impostor syndrome, gambling mentality, and even brain fog.

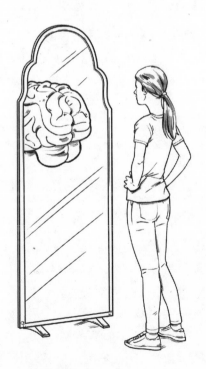

You have uncovered many of the brain's secrets in this book so far. Now follow me down a path that's part useful conjecture and part wisdom to discover advanced brainhacks that can control us, our actions, luck, and success itself.

32 | Memory and Mirror: Status, Identity, and the Reason for Emotions

> Status is to humans what water is to fish; we don't think about
> it, but it affects everything.
>
> **—Keith Johnstone**

I believe many of our mental traits we think are intrinsic like self-esteem, confidence, grit, and identity are essentially just the act of memorizing information and comparing it to other information. This is the basis of a very simple model of the brain I use. Any similarity to any other theory or idea is coincidental, and I haven't proven it . . . *yet*, so decide for yourself if the model helps you.

I thought of this idea after teaching brain training for decades. Something clicked when I applied my memory theory to other brain functions, all driven at their core by emotion. The current popular thinking on emotions is that they are distinct (in form and function) from logic and memory. But what if we have misunderstood the nature and purpose of emotions? I believe it's been under our noses the whole time. Feelings (everything from how you feel about gummies to guns) are just a type of memory. I don't mean that feelings make us remember things. I mean that every feeling you have ever felt is an association—a memory link—that your brain created to help you navigate the world.

BRAIN ASSIGNS A VALUE

As you go through life, your brain associates feelings with everything you see, hear, and think to help you make decisions. We know there are strong and weak feelings; in therapy, people are often asked to rank feelings in order of significance and often result in dozens of levels of emotion. Imagine that that is just your brain giving an experience a number value.

Let's say the first time you ever ate a hamburger, your brain associated the feeling of deliciousness at a level four out of five. Later, you try a pizza for the first time, and it scores five out of five. Later, when your friend asks you which one you prefer to eat, you would choose the pizza because it *feels* better, though you have no logical idea why. In reality, your brain scored it higher, and the decision was entirely subconscious. This is a huge oversimplification, but there is a medical condition that supports this idea that emotions exist primarily to help us make decisions.

Dr. Antonio Damasio studied a specific type of brain damage that removed a patient's ability to feel emotions. Without the ability to feel anything, you might think these people would be logical and decisive, right? Wrong. Their biggest challenge wasn't with relationships or social interaction. Rather, when they lost emotions, they lost the ability to make even the simplest of decisions.

After a session, Dr. Damasio would ask them when they would like to come in again: Tuesday or Thursday. They would struggle, unable to pick because neither day *felt* different from the other. This suggests that emotions aren't the opposite of logic; they're a logical shortcut. You have a feeling for everything you encounter, from the person who creeps you out on the bus to the keychain you think is cute but not as cute as the purple one. Feelings are like little emotional tags attached to everything we experience, so if you ever have to make a quick choice between them, you can do it. It's a genius way to make decisions quickly without processing all of the details every time. It's nature's timesaver. (I think this concept alone could be powerful if applied to an AI model.)

Emotional Reactions

When our emotions get the best of us, it's usually because we have two or more very strong feelings (memories about a subject) that are competing. Like the feeling of loving a pet versus the feeling of losing it. The pain is the brain trying to make sense of something that will never make sense.

Imagine for a moment that you had to go through an intricate, logic-based thought process every time you chose what to eat for lunch. Forget that. Instead, you *feel* like having a pizza, so you have it.

EMOTIONS DECIDE, LOGIC JUSTIFIES

Advertisers and politicians know that decisions are made with emotions, not logic. Indeed, humans make nearly all buying and voting decisions based on emotions, and then later justify them with logic.

I have been hired by companies to teach salespeople. We would raise sales by teaching them how to memorize customers' names and recall product information. This made the customer *feel* like they are not just a number and are working with an expert. This is an honest way to achieve more sales, but we all know dishonest marketing that exploits emotions and manipulates people. These tactics only work because decisions are made via emotions. There is no money in appealing to logic.

Fight Back with Logic Hack

To fight back against the manipulation of your emotions by others, start to get into the habit of making decisions with logic. Anyone can do this at any time, but it needs continuous effort. Next time you have a decision, try writing down on paper the pros and cons of the decision instead of going with feelings. It takes practice.

So far, this makes sense when applied to small things. But who cares why we order pizza over hamburgers? You need to know why your emotions go crazy when someone cuts you off or why people will be willing to fight, kill, and die for emotional reasons. Emotions can feel like a kind of temporary insanity or the ultimate reward. How can all of these situations come from a mnemonic mechanism geared to make quick decisions?

To understand this, we have to go back to the environment this emotional mechanism is suited to. *Nature.* Remember the hunter-gatherer story from before? You may recall our memory is suited to help us survive by remembering where a predator or a food source is. But if you only avoided dangers that you directly encountered, you wouldn't last long. So, your brain also uses thousands of tiny memories to attach to every trait of the food or danger you want to pay attention to. So, the hunter-gatherer doesn't just remember to look out for crocodiles in that one watering hole you saw them in as a kid, but to be wary of every place that is similar because small ponds of still water *feel* dangerous. They don't just remember to avoid eating that one red poisonous berry; now, all red berries are suspect.

Now take this amazing tool for survival in the wild and put it in modern life. That person who cut you off in traffic is threatening your life by blocking you from your hunting grounds, and that tweet that made fun of your hat makes it feel like you could be kicked out of your tribe. So, that emotional overreaction makes sense when you understand that the brain's mirror compares these things to very dire results because of our evolutionary history.

Here is the useful part. First, by being aware that emotions are just memory connections that often misfire or don't apply to modern life, you can change how you react to them. Second, using this approach, you can change many traits previously thought immutable with nothing more than brainhacks.

HACK BAGGAGE

A hundred thousand years ago, feelings were simple. They helped guide us. We would look at two roads diverging in the woods, and our subconscious would compare it to past experiences, giving us the feeling to go in the right direction. But our ancestors' lives would hardly change as they grew up, so the old lessons learned as a kid were useful as adults. Feelings were a good guide. Today's rate of change means that feelings we experienced ten years ago aren't a good guide to life now, and that conflict causes us a lot of our suffering. Start hacking away at this by being aware of old patterns.

Old Patterns Hack

Next time you feel strong emotions, ask yourself if this is an old pattern repeating from your past. As you learn how to hack these emotions, start editing this baggage. Awareness is the first step.

For example, we think self-esteem is this complex, immutable trait. I believe it's simply a legion of simple connections we have made about ourselves rolled into one concept. But these decisions were often made a long time ago, and times have changed. As we encounter situations, our current feelings conflict with older ones, causing an emotional reaction.

Everyone has things they like and don't like about themselves. This is normal, and emotions are simply your brain's way of keeping score. When you run a mile, your brain adds a number to the athletic column; when you get rejected by your crush, it subtracts from your charisma.

Your brain compares these data points with each other internally and externally with the wider world in a constant attempt to see where you fit into your peer group. This is what we call status. All these data points can be hacked and changed with new stimuli, but only by taking charge of them can we end the suffering of internal conflict.

STRONG EMOTIONS

Have you ever had a good cry that helped you make a decision or think about a problem differently? Strong emotional reactions come from a clash between two or more feelings. I once had a trusted friend who betrayed me. I felt hurt and angry. In the moment, I had to reconcile two opposing ideas: how I felt about my friend and how I felt about the betrayal. I think your brain creates strong emotional reactions to help decide which emotion in the conflict is true. It's like a computer short-circuiting; it can't decide how to react. For example, I see myself as very athletic, so when I gained weight, I got upset. How I *felt* about myself was at odds with reality.

The clash between two brain connections will cause a reaction—negative, like sadness and depression, or positive, like motivation and drive to exercise. Either way, I want you to understand that how you feel is just a connection in the brain, and it can be changed to eliminate your struggle. The world isn't against you. Your brain does not hate you. You're not broken.

Once we assume this is the way emotions work in the brain, so many other things make sense, like how social media influences us. Your brain is still the same as that of the ancient hunter-gatherer whose peer group consisted of twenty people in a small village. But now, thanks to social media and the twenty-four-hour news cycle, your peer group is the entire world. So, you are comparing your average day to mankind's best-filtered photos.

If you were put down a lot as a kid like I was, then the memory attached to self-worth is low. So, you have a low idea of how much money you deserve. But you could also have had other experiences later in life where you feel you deserve a raise. So then, the internal clash becomes emotionally hard to bear and you feel impostor syndrome. (Of course, there are external factors relating to success too. Life is tough, but it's even tougher when your emotions fight you.)

Emotional Reaction Brainhack

Next time, try to look objectively at emotional reactions and see if they still serve you. Our biggest internal problems come when these emotional states clash. When our emotions get the best of us, we find it helpful to think of them as a connection that is illogical.

I spent a few weeks working on this and didn't realize how big a difference it made in my life until one day, when I drove a friend to the airport. I felt something shift.

I love doing little favors for friends, and I am asked to give people a ride or advice all the time. Every time they thanked me, I would say, "It was nothing." It was my way of minimizing what I did.

This time, I pulled up to the airport to drop my friend off, and they thanked me as usual, and I almost said, "it was nothing," but I stopped just before the words came out. From the outside, it looked weird, like I rebooted mid-sentence, and maybe I did. The words we use have power.

I realized that I kept saying that it was nothing, and for the first time, I couldn't say it because I valued my effort and time more than before. The words didn't fit anymore. I still loved to help others, but it wasn't nothing. It was a big deal. I had a lot of work to do, and I helped this friend by giving him a ride. I would only get this thank you in return, and I'd always push it away. It reminded me of all the times I was told I was stupid or worthless growing up.

This hack *did* change my bank account. I turned my memory seminar into a product. I sold over one hundred thousand copies worldwide in a short period of time, making me an international best-selling author. Today, I regularly speak to businesses for over ten thousand dollars (though my rate for colleges is much lower, by choice). So yes, it changes your ledger.

But this brainhack is about more than just making money. It's about how you are valued in this world.

I would keep doing the mental training to raise how much I felt I deserve in life. There would be a knock-on effect. Yes, it can lead to making more money, but it also helps with relationships. You can't truly love until you feel you deserve it yourself, and when your head is full of self-hate, you can ruin a great relationship.

When you *do* value yourself, you take care of yourself. The world seems to look different. I feel a little taller, calmer, and more deserving.

At the airport drop-off, it confused my friend to see me looking off into space, so he interrupted my train of thought as he grabbed his bags, ready to leave. "Dave," he said, "thanks for this ride. I really appreciate this, man."

"You're welcome," I said and meant it.

CHAPTER **SUMMARY**

- As you go through life, your brain assigns values to everything you encounter. These values help us make quicker decisions when choosing between two options. In fact, the data shows that people make most of their decisions this way.
- Our emotional reactions happen when there is a major conflict between different values for the same thing, like being in love but fearing the other person doesn't feel the same.
- People who want to manipulate you will try to trigger your emotions. Fight back with logic and reason.
- Now that you are aware of your brain's tendency to assign values, take charge of the process by thinking about what you want and value. Look for conflicts in your baggage and decide to change your values. This is the start. Visualizing the end result you want helps make the change.

33 | You Win Some...

> You are not poor. Poor is a mentality. It's a mentality that very few
> people ever recover from. Don't you forget it, son. You are *broke*.
> **—Dave Chappelle (recounting advice from**
> **his father that changed his life)**

I stared at him knowing I was right. This man before me wore an old suit
and a pair of thick black plastic-rimmed glasses and was pretending to
eat while looking around with a goofy grin.

He was Herb! No one would dress like this on purpose in a Burger King!

This is the story of how Herb taught me about the mental thermostat, which is the invisible setting in our brain that determines how much
money, love, or success we feel we deserve. It can motivate but also create
impostor syndrome and self-sabotage.

It was 1985, and Burger King stores held a contest where anyone could
win $5,000 if they spotted Herb in their stores. All they had to do was walk
up to him and say a magic phrase.

At the time, Burger King was being destroyed by a Wendy's commercial featuring three old ladies poking at a big bun with a tiny hamburger
in it (making fun of other chains), asking, "Where's the beef?" This catch-
phrase became the most popular saying in existence for years. So, Wendy's

put the slogan on hats, shirts, frisbees, sold an entire Milton Bradley board game, and released an album.

Think about that for a second. This ad campaign was so successful, they sold an entire music album with these ninety-year-old ladies making songs about the beef slogan! Even politicians used the phrase to attack their opponent's lack of substance. You haven't lived until you've seen a presidential candidate ask their opponent, "Where's the beef?"

To counter this, Burger King created one of the stupidest ad campaigns in history: the Where's Herb? contest.

It was the eighties, and I was just ten.

I'm reaching back in time for this hack because the lesson I learned back then only came to make sense when I was an adult. Here, you will learn how to hack self-esteem, confidence, and more. It may be the most impactful hack in this entire book.

Herb always looked like he'd dressed in the dark. He was a combination of Herb Tarlek from WKRP and the perfect '80s nerd. The '80s were obsessed with nerds the same way comic geeks took over the 2000s.

This campaign was like playing *Where's Waldo?* with a chance to win cash when you spotted this secret eater in a restaurant.

And I was staring at him. I was sure of it.

(Nearly every reference in this chapter makes me feel old.)

I pointed to him and whispered to my mom, "That's him. That's Herb!" She knew about the campaign, but she said not to worry about it and to just keep eating.

I pressed, having only eaten a few fries so far. I wasn't going to let hydrogenated-vegetable-oil-fried goodies distract me from my potential payday. I was already counting the money in my head.

My dad said, "Stop it. Don't embarrass us."

I became annoyingly persistent, not letting it go. Eventually, my mom gave in and walked over to talk to him.

This was around the time I was learning lipreading, and I liked to practice it in public. Now, I thought it would pay off. I could follow their conversation word for word.

Mom: "Hi, can I ask you something?"

Herb: "Sure."

Mom: "You're Herb, aren't you?"

Herb: "Yes, I am."

My heart stopped. He had unmistakably replied in the affirmative. She just had to say the secret phrase, and we would win $5,000.

"I thought so. Thank you," Mom said. Then, she walked away without a word. I nearly fainted. What was happening?

When my mother got back to the table, she wanted to go. I protested.

My dad shook his head. "If he was Herb, your mother would have said the phrase. Now let's go."

Dumbfounded, I searched their faces for clues about what the heck was happening. To this day, I'm still surprised by the look on their faces. Neither disbelief nor anger with me for being annoying.

Instead, they looked afraid.

I was dragged to the car, as I asked my mother. "He said yes, didn't he, Mom? I could read your lips."

She was stoic, saying nothing.

Only when the truck started to swim with the stream of traffic she spoke. "Yes, it was Herb."

"Dad, turn around. You heard it yourself. It was Herb!!" I explained, feeling like a lawyer winning a case.

He hardened his face and said, "There's no such thing as free money."

At the time, I thought it was the most idiotic phrase in the world because there was clearly free money sitting there waiting for us at that Burger King. We could really use the money too.

THE MENTAL THERMOSTAT CONCEPT

My parents reacted that way because of how the brain connects our income to our self-worth. The most powerful emotional connections we make are to our own ego or sense of self. We know the brain attaches values to things to create emotions. The mental thermostat is an enforcement mechanism that uses chemistry to reward or punish us to stay near the range we feel we deserve.

It will calculate how strong or smart we are and then rank us with others. But interestingly, if an experience challenges the order of the hierarchy, people don't change their self-esteem; they actually fight to enforce their imaginary beliefs, even if it means running away from free money.

It could be a raise, promotion, feeling loved, or a standing ovation. We get what we feel we deserve, and if we don't feel we deserve it, we will continue to self-sabotage or develop impostor syndrome, ruining the experience. That's what caused my parents to leave that day, and it's what caused my rut after the Guinness record. But that was just the start.

I thought about the Where's Herb? incident for years and judged my parents until I did the exact same thing.

* * *

And now back to the future (another '80s reference)! In my twenties, I was making a great living doing seminars for local real estate offices, schools, and the public. Parents and students were so happy with the results that they recommended me to a local college. I was even willing to cut my fee down to make it happen. Anything to help reach students who were struggling like me.

The college had a budget for outside speakers, and we talked about a fee of $1,000 for my talk—which is low for this kind of thing. But they wanted to negotiate even further. I would find out later that other speakers were given as much as five to ten thousand for talks like this, but they didn't think I was worth it, and maybe I didn't either.

I gave in, wanting to reach the students more than make a payday. I suggested I would take all the risks and offer the class if the college agreed to pay per student. I asked for only $20 per student, and half would be paid by the students themselves. This was a tremendous risk, because I could lose money after my expenses. They were still skeptical that the students would be interested at all, so I doubled down, saying that I would do the class no matter how few showed up. Even with two students, I could still teach them my secrets. I wasn't the best negotiator, but I knew students were struggling. I see the same thing at every college and university I go to. Students who did well in high school are struggling because they didn't learn how their brains work. Academic workload is listed as the number one reason for dropping out.

I was also used to this kind of elitism from educational institutes. Businesses would bring me in and take advantage of my insights, but even my offers to volunteer for schools were met with negativity. It made sense on one level. After all, I was going to an institute of higher learning to teach how to learn, and they were skeptical. They didn't like to be taught how to teach by a twentysomething.

The administrator dismissed my pay-per-student suggestion. He said, "If students wanted to learn study skills, there are already a lot of resources on campus."

I was used to being underestimated, but I should have been more worried about success, not failure.

"Just so you know," the administrator said, "in the past, students didn't pay for anything. We tried to get them to pay $5 for food during orientation, but they already expect so much included in tuition."

A week later, hundreds of students had signed up.

It was the most satisfying program I had taught up to that point. These students needed help, asked brilliant questions, and did all the exercises diligently. The results were significant too. I have letters and emails from students who said that just one session turned around their studies. They were about to quit because they were failing, and the study skills allowed them to graduate. This led to me doing hundreds of talks helping students around the world.

According to the deal, I calculated that the school owed me over ten thousand, but they only paid *four* thousand. Nonetheless, I actually walked away from that experience feeling good because I wasn't doing it for the money. I knew I had made an impact.

Growing up, my family pinched pennies and relied on charity to get toys during the holidays. We shopped at garage sales. After I deposited the money in the bank, my joy turned to dread. Over the next week, I fell into a deep depression, but not for the reason you may think. It was a feeling of not deserving to be comfortable. I had grown up struggling financially, and even as an entrepreneur I lived sale to sale. So, when I had more money than I needed, it felt like I did something wrong. This is the mental thermostat at work.

THE CURSE OF THE LOTTERY

Anyone can experience this. A good example of the mental thermostat is the curse of the lottery. Within three years, most lottery winners are broke and in debt, many even addicted to drugs and regretting the day they won that money. The mental thermostat also applies to very confident people. You can be highly skilled, famous, and at the top of your field, but still have a brain that will knock you down to the financial level it thinks you should be at. Take professional athletes, for instance. According to research, a large number of pro athletes come from poor backgrounds and even after getting millions of dollars in contracts along with high praise and love from fans, three years after they retire, many are broke. Sound familiar?

Countless studies have also shown this phenomenon at play with lesser amounts of money. Everything from lawsuit payouts to pay raises, scholarships to welfare. This phenomenon of self-worth is complex and goes beyond money. In our relationships, the belief that a partner is high above us in social status can sabotage the relationship because we don't believe we deserve their love.

A couple weeks after the seminar in the college, I was deeply depressed. I could barely get out of bed to wash. I was stuck in a vicious cycle: self-hatred for achieving financial success, leading to a lack of action, then more self-loathing due to my failure to act. I'm embarrassed that it only took four thousand dollars to do this to me when today I sign deals for fifty thousand dollars at a time without blinking. But the dollar amount isn't the point. Depression and self-esteem aren't logical. You may have never experienced this feeling of depression before. It wasn't the amount of money in the bank that did it, but the idea that I thought of myself as a person who always struggled. For the first time, I was fine and that made me not fine. I'm telling this story to show that even financial stability can trigger depression if your brain is wired wrong. For others, it could be love, being shown respect, being given responsibility, or being put on center stage.

I never once believed consciously that I should be depressed, but my logic wasn't in charge. I would love to say I figured out a brainhack in a couple of weeks and changed everything without any further missteps, but this isn't so simple. Eventually, I spent the money and dipped into debt a bit. Once I was broke again, the drive to make money came back, and the depression left.

I learned that just giving a man a fish isn't enough—and neither is teaching him to fish. People need to believe they *deserve* the fish.

Thermostat Hack

So, your brain brings together thousands of different data points to decide where you fit in the social hierarchy. This position is enforced with chemical rewards and punishments in your nervous system. This system is one of the oldest functions in our evolutionary history. It goes back nearly half a billion years. We can't stop our brain from enforcing its belief with this chemical system. But we can change the memories it uses as a measure.

Try this:

Step One: Write down on paper what you want your mental thermostat to be. I don't know your situation, but everyone wants something they don't feel they deserve. Write down your challenge.

Step Two: Visualize yourself doing what you desire successfully over and over. Visualization is similar to, but not the same as, meditation. You don't need to be in a trance or take much time.

For example, this could be done in sixty seconds while you brush your teeth.

Step Three: Ask questions to make your visualizations more powerful. Questions focus the brain and make stronger scenes. Don't just imagine a big house, ask yourself what the door looks like; then, ask your brain to pick the tile floor and place the furniture. Finally, ask yourself "Where is the couch?" and "What color are the walls?" Let your mind paint the picture, and it will stick much more. This makes it feel real, and feelings are what we are going for here.

Step Four: Social proof helps. After you have painted a picture of what you want, visualize others saying you deserve this success. Social cues count for more in value changes than our own opinion. Imagine loved ones being impressed and showing their support.

Step Five: Repeat as necessary (and it *is* necessary). At first, some of these exercises will make you feel like a fraud and even hate yourself for doing it. This is the clash between the image and the lack of self-esteem you have now. Over time, visualize these images again and again. Soon, you will feel the difference—and not even recognize the old you.

Note: You may really struggle making these images at first. It could be from a lack of practice visualizing, or you really can't imagine some of the positive things you want. This is normal. Your new brain won't be built in a day. Start with small things you can imagine and do it every day. Over time, you will get better and better.

Keep doing it, and positive mental images will pile up, replacing the negative ones. You've probably received thousands of negative messages in your life to feel the way you do now. Hence, you need to replace them with thousands of positive ones. Keep going. Make a calendar, and do it twice a day for a month. Even after you feel better, keep going. Lock it in, because I can tell you from experience, the feelings will come back if you aren't thorough.

The goal is to enjoy the freedom of being a self-made person, having the ability to erase and rewrite your personal baggage. Of course, this is easier said than done, but the reward is worth it. If you want more help, go to brainhackers.com for support, and give feedback about what has worked for you.

CHAPTER **SUMMARY**

- The Mental Thermostat Concept states that there is a force in our nervous system that uses chemical rewards and punishments to motivate us to stick within a predetermined status range. Things like how much money we can make, how much love and support we can accept, and more are all determined by this mechanism that dates back nearly half a billion years in our history. We can't stop this reward system, but we can change the setting.
- The mental thermostat is so powerful it will make us ruin our lives if we come into a windfall. The majority of people who win money or get major sports contracts are broke within three years due to this problem. Giving others money will not help improve lives unless their brain believes they deserve it.
- To change your thermostat setting, visualize the person you want to be over and over. The thermostat also reacts to social cues so imagine your friends, family, and even strangers rooting for you in these images. Then repeat this a lot. We get so many negative messages thrown at us regularly that we need a lot to counter them.

34 | Is Success Luck or Hard Work?

You win battles by knowing the enemy's timing, and using a timing which the enemy does not expect.

—**Miyamoto Musashi (known as Japan's greatest swordsman)**

After resetting the mental thermostat, we need a lucky break. But what if I told you luck is actually a combination of strategy and brainhacks?

First, let's answer the question: Is success the result of luck or hard work? This debate has raged on for centuries. The "luck" believers make an emotional appeal to convince us the game is rigged and people with billions of dollars or model good looks are simply born into success, ignoring their contribution to the world.

The "hard work" group points to data showing that nearly every success started as a failure, and those who work hard are usually much better off in life, ignoring the fact that some start at a different place than others. Then, the luckists show that a small group of families or companies control almost all the wealth. But the workists show that these families were different from those in control just thirty years ago, and over time, the ones on top change often, meaning it's mostly a meritocracy.

Claims have been made that 70% of wealth is inherited. But, at the same time, another study says that only 30% of family wealth survives for one generation.

I believe this is a false debate, because we are asking the wrong question.

Luck is not what we have been told it is. It's not random. To hack luck, we first have to hack the brain to eliminate the gambling mentality that is inherent in all of us. Then, replace it with a mindset based on game theory. Because the type of luck we are talking about is not chance at all; for the most part, luck is . . . *timing*.

If a person walking down the street is suddenly hit by an air-conditioning unit falling from ten stories above, we would all think he was unlucky. But if that unit narrowly misses him, then he's lucky, right? The variable is time. Everyone says that luck means being in the right place at the right time. But when you replace the concept of "good luck" with the concept of "good timing," it makes more sense why some people seem to get more of it than others. Timing is something we can have some control over.

Release a new product right when the market wants it, and that's lucky. On the other hand, release it too late or too early, and that's bad luck. Go into school for a job that's in demand, and you're lucky enough to find a job after graduating.

It's also important to mention that most of the time, you can't control timing. Try picking stocks or predicting the market, and at some point, you will be slapped down. Sure, you'll be called a genius for getting in on Bitcoin when it's low. Or you might follow the same instincts right on another speculation and lose everything. But through it all, there are strategies based on math and game theory that can give you an advantage.

Before we master these strategies, though, we need to purge ourselves of the curse of the gamblers' mindset . . . something I learned by card counting.

* * *

I never intended to be a card counter. I was almost thirty, and at this point in my life, I was teaching memory at live events, speaking at colleges, and doing a lot of media interviews. I was good at speaking to the media, thanks to the help of some mentors. I was able to turn these interviews into online traffic and book sales, making my book a best seller.

In these interviews, though, there was one question I was asked over and over that I had no answer for: "Can you count cards?"

One time in the early 2000s, I was on *The Jeff and Jer Show* in San Diego. Dave Grohl from the Foo Fighters was on just before me. It was the big leagues. When they asked if I could count cards, I was embarrassed, but that week I had made nearly two hundred thousand dollars in sales, so this thought went to the back burner. Until my old friend Scott said, "I heard the show. Good job, man, but you stumbled a bit when he asked about card counting."

I told him, "I get asked that question all the time, and it gets annoying."

"You gotta think like a showman," he said, flashing a smile and switching into his magician stage persona. "Give the people what they want and tempt them with a dream. That's what magic is all about."

"I'm not a magician. I'm an educator," I replied with a shake of my head. "I want to be taken seriously."

"You are a lot of things, but when you are on a radio or TV show, you are an entertainer—plus, you're one of the smartest guys I know. If you wanted to, you could master card counting and have a great story to tell. People pay attention to the guy with the best story." He had a point.

So, after looking at all the credible card counting systems, I used a basic version of one from the book *Playing Blackjack as a Business*. If you want to count cards, I suggest you begin and end with that book.

I practiced at home until I was good enough to play and win. Scott did the training along with me and got good at counting himself.

THE GAMBLER'S MENTALITY

The gambler's mentality is a complex problem big enough to fill a book itself. A major part of it is an unintended consequence of the visualization principle. Remember that feeling the last time you thought you left the stove on? What triggered that feeling was probably a stray thought about the possibility. Then once you visualized it, your brain thinks it actually happened and you can't let it go unless you check. In the same way, when you place a bet, you visualize winning and then can't get it out of your head. This is the visualization principle working against you.

This is why instincts about winning are almost always wrong. These feelings lead us to action, and we buy a lottery ticket or bet on a game. We do this in other areas too. Say for example you are dating someone, and you imagine it going badly because of low self-esteem or a previous bad experience. Your brain visualizes that image and thus thinks it has already gone bad, giving you the feeling of dread about the relationship. If you believe it, then you start to make the relationship implode as a self-fulfilling prophecy. This only reinforces the myth that your emotions are good at predicting the future—when really, they helped create it.

The hack for this is simple.

Gambler's Mentality Hack

Stop imagining worst- and best-case scenarios, and do the math. Any time you are in a defeatist or gambler's mindset, the situation is likely not that dire or that great. Stop and think.

This reminds me of when a friend told me they thought the whole world was out to get them and everyone hated them. I said that that was crazy; the vast majority of the world doesn't care about you enough to hate you. This broke the pattern and got a laugh. Every once in a while, we need to be reminded that nothing is as bad or good as it feels. Stop and do a little math.

THE LAW OF MULTIPLE TRIES

The rules of blackjack are set up so you lose a little more often than you win. But by keeping track of the ratio of high cards to low cards, you can predict when you will win and lose.

Low cards like two to six add one point to the count, and high cards like ten and face cards are minus one. (Depending on the system, aces and fives might be counted separately, but that's a long story.) Math tells us ten cards are more likely to help me win, and low cards help the dealer. By tracking how many high and low cards have been played, we know the chances of the cards we want coming out of the shoe. (A shoe is what they call the stack of playing cards used in the game.)

This only gives counters about a 2% chance of success above the house. But we can predict when that 2% chance will happen and bet more, making our winnings much higher. This game is a lot like life itself. Although it looks like the odds of any major project, business, job interview, or life plan will fail, when you look at it over the long term, you can set things up to always succeed with the law of multiple tries.

Card counting and game theory work on the idea that there are multiple rounds to most games. If there is only one roll of the dice, then it's all about chance, but the more tries you get at a game, the more strategy plays a role. Counting through a 6–8 deck shoe gives me time to beat the game by predicting the chances of good cards being dealt.

Bring this mindset into the game of life, and the math guarantees success. Often, we give up after getting rejected or disappointed a couple of times. But every story of success from your favorite musician to famous inventions have hundreds of failures before success comes. In blackjack, I know I will lose many hands in a row, so I bet the lowest possible to minimize the loss, and then when I start to win, I bet much more, covering my losses and making a profit.

The same strategy works for most things in life. If you can attempt something with no real cost of failure, like my Guinness record attempt for example, then you can try as many times as you want. You only need to succeed once, and it pays for every failure and much more.

* * *

In high school, I told my guidance counselor that I wanted to run a business. She tried to convince me to do anything else, and said that only one in ten businesses succeed.

"You really think it's that high?" I replied. "That makes it much easier than I thought. All I have to do is try ten times, and I'm guaranteed to succeed."

She just stared at me not knowing what to say. It just seemed logical to me that if I didn't stop trying, then I would eventually succeed.

If you have ever seen a person who is not smart or talented running an organization and wonder why, you may think they were born into the business or somehow got lucky. The truth is that, in nearly every example, you'll find out they just never stopped trying until they succeeded.

This is sometimes called making your own luck. If you flip a coin often enough, it will be heads.

I recently read a book that tried to argue that luck plays a higher role in success than previously thought. Those who succeed believe they are special and skilled because of survivorship bias. All the examples they gave, however, were situations where there was only one chance to win a game. Like becoming an astronaut or playing major league sports. This was dishonest and misleading because math shows us that nearly any game with infinite tries can be beaten, and life is such a game. You haven't lost until you give up or die. Every success story is full of hundreds of tries to make a thing work before the one time it did.

Saying "don't give up" is not enough, though. Try this mindset: Make it your job to try and become the person you want to be. Wake up every day trying and possibly failing. Don't even count the failures, just make the effort your full-time job. If you get this mindset, you are guaranteed to succeed.

CHAPTER **SUMMARY**

- Luck is not just about randomness. When we are talking about success in life, luck is usually a matter of timing.
- Counting showed me that luck is influenced by strategy, but only when it's a game with multiple tries. The good news is that nearly every area of life gives us the opportunity for multiple attempts.
- Lose the Gambler's Mentality. Our brains are geared to gamble. Wanting success or money alone isn't the problem. It's the lack of seeing the risk in the process. Hack this by asking yourself: *What could I lose?*

35 | Mind Over Luck

I walked into the casino for the first time, ready to play. I had practiced counting the cards while watching the tables for a while, confident I could keep up with the speed, and now it was time to make some money.

Sitting down, I gave the dealer a few hundred and got my chips, placing the minimum bet on the table as the new shoe's first cards were dealt. Different tables use larger shoes of six to eight decks, and others advertise that only one deck is used.

As the dealer dealt out two cards, each face-up, she dealt herself two leaving one up and one hidden. Using a tiny mirror on the table, she checked if the face-down card was an ace. (That would have meant she won blackjack and would have to deal again.) It wasn't, so the game was on.

I had fourteen and the dealer had seven. The chances were less than 26% that the dealer would bust and 74% that the dealer would get between 17 and 21 So, I hit. I got seventeen and stayed. The dealer got twenty, and I lost. But the count was going my way. After a few more hands, the count was above seven, so I doubled my bet. I won and doubled again (a common gambler move, so it didn't look suspicious). I won again, but after a lot of ten cards, the count went negative, so I left to another table. I kept this up for an hour, and then left.

I didn't want to get caught, so I bounced around from casino to casino, never playing for more than an hour at a time in any one place. This was my job for about a year, moving through different casinos and following my rules. I would increase my bet when the count was high and sometimes wait till my first winning hand. To an outside observer, it would look as though I had a hunch.

I won't go in-depth on all the nuances of blackjack, card counting, and the system I used versus other methods. That would take a book of its own. Good thing I already wrote an ebook on the subject! It's available for download on brainhackers.com.

The system worked, and the money came in. I was regularly walking around with tens of thousands of dollars in cash and chips. When you have that much cash, you tend to spend it, so I saw every show from Penn and Teller to Cirque du Soleil and everything with the word *revue*. I still flew home from Las Vegas each time with thousands of dollars from the weekend's efforts. It was an exciting time.

THE LUCK MINDSET

Now that we can avoid the gambler's mindset, let's focus on the luck mindset. The following are a series of small hacks and strategies that maximize your luck and timing. In the process of reading through these hacks, you will see that many of the traits we associate with luck are actually within our control. Think of these all under the category of developing a mindset of luck as a skill, not a gift.

Luck Mindset Brainhacks

Just Beat the Dealer

One brainhack is a way to think about success. For example, the game appears simple at first. The goal is to reach twenty-one without going over, right? Actually, no. The casino wants you to try for twenty-one because if you try, you will fail a lot more often than if you try for the real goal of the game, which is to beat the dealer . . . something that's much easier to do.

Think about that as a metaphor. How often are we aiming at the wrong goal or trying to reach perfection when winning is simpler than we are making it?

The Luck of Patience

Those who appear lucky in life often have the discipline to wait for the right time to act. The best plan is to decide what you want to achieve, and then wait for the deal to show up. From houses to job offers, waiting for the right deal brings good fortune. I learned this firsthand waiting for the cards to turn. One of the biggest lessons I learned from counting cards was money management—knowing when to hold 'em and when to bet. It's tempting to bet more when you feel hot, but follow the math and be patient. The key is to have rules set up in advance that you follow so you don't get caught up in the moment.

Model Success

Instead of being jealous, make a study of others in the field or project you want success in. Chances are they are doing something no one else is. Model them and you will find the same luck transfers to you. It seems the more I learn, the luckier I get.

Supply and Demand

Find out what you are good at that others struggle with. I started learning brainhacks to solve my own problems, only to discover others wanted to know these secrets too. Decades later, it's still in demand. Get where you want to go by giving others what they want, but make sure your skills and what you offer are what people want.

Macro Matches Micro

The principle of fractal mathematics is that the large scale will match the small scale if they are acted on by the same forces. It's true. A small stretch of beach has a similar jagged pattern to the entire coastline it's a part of. In the same way, it's smart to test the waters in a small environment, then scale up. Like a comedian who tests their jokes in a small club to make sure people laugh before using them on a TV special, or a job applicant who does mock interviews with friends before applying. I did this with card counting, testing my system with low stakes before scaling up. We do the same with marketing.

The Real Win-Win

When people hear the term "win-win," they think of a deal that benefits both parties. That's a nice sentiment, but you are probably more at risk of being taken advantage of in life if you don't look out for your own interests first. This hack is about making a win-win strategy that benefits you if it works and also if it fails. Think of how a bank works. You borrow money, and they get interest, but if you don't pay, they own the house. They win no matter what.

Often, we set up plans that place ourselves in the martyr position. From the outside, it just looks like you are unlucky, but really, you took a bad deal.

This is also the strategy of Warren Buffett. He would find undervalued companies to invest in. If they grew, he would make a profit, but if they went bankrupt, he could recoup his loss when they sell off assets. Simple, right? But due to the gambling mentality, 90% of investing is speculation. That's gambling, not investing. It's about more than investing, though. I have a clause in my speaking contract that guarantees me half pay if the event is canceled, for example. Think about how you could protect yourself in a worst-case scenario.

> ### Extend Trend Lines
>
> There was a book written in 1994 titled *The World in 2020* by Hamish McRae. This book was more correct in its future predictions than nearly any other source I could find. What was the secret? All the author did was make charts of trends that were happening, then extend them further. Many predictions were spot on, from oil prices to housing crashes, cultural issues, and climate change. The key is that he let go of all dogma and just looked at charts and extended them into the future. You can do this to predict your career and future plans. It's not speculation, it's math.

ALL GOOD THINGS COME TO AN END

My card counting run stopped one day at Harrah's Casino. It's known for blackjack, and it was my favorite at the time. I was wearing the counter's uniform, a baseball cap and glasses with no prescription. I was up about ten grand and felt cocky. I wasn't waiting to win a hand before doubling the bet, and I was obvious about looking at the cards to the point where the dealer made a joke about counting. I was basically breaking all my rules by getting cocky.

I was dealt two tens with a thousand dollar bet on the table, and the count was still high. I split. This is an option when you get a pair. One hand becomes two. I separated each card and placed a second thousand in chips on the table, receiving two more cards. Both tens.

The dealer busted, and I collected. Focused on the chips, I didn't notice two guys in dark suits standing behind me. I was about to place another bet when the look on the dealer's face stopped me. A huge hand landed on my shoulder with a thud and turned me around.

"Could you come with us, please, sir?" the man in black said.

I had read about this but hadn't experienced it yet. This was casino security. They are there to be intimidating, but they had no legal authority.

I was surprised he even touched me because situations like these can devolve into lawsuits.

They wanted to do what was called "backrooming." It's exactly as creepy as it sounds. The casino security will take you into a backroom and take your picture and fingerprints and generally intimidate you. They have no legal right to do this because card counting is not illegal, but they hope you don't know that. They also want your ID so the IRS can harass you and even detectives can follow you.

I had to think fast and talk faster. So, I pretended they were here to offer me a perk or comp (this is when a hotel gives a player something to encourage them to keep gambling). "Hey guys, I'm actually staying at another hotel, so I don't need comps here," I said, collecting my chips in shaking hands. "Give any bonuses to another person. I just realized I have to get going."

If looks could kill, theirs would have incinerated me. But I kept telling myself they couldn't touch me. They were standing between me and the exit, though. So, I did an awkward sideways shuffle around them as I thanked them for the comp offers, making sure not to touch them at all. Once free, I walked to the exit. I felt like a rope or hook would grab me and pull me back in, but none came. Casinos want to spread the myth that counting is wrong or dishonest. But at one point in time, the casinos were even forbidden from kicking out counters. They will make your life hell if you're caught, though.

I was spooked and laid low for a while. I looked back at that time and noticed that while I focused on card counting, my core business didn't grow. Running around with a lot of cash wasn't good for me, and I didn't really save any. I didn't end up with much to show for my efforts. Vegas has a way to get your money by game or by vice. I did manage to confirm that I wasn't put on any counting list, so I would not be harassed. But what about next time?

Although I know counters that have done well, many professional gamblers never get to retire and are always moving from score to score. So, it's not a long-term strategy for success.

After several months of focusing on my memory business, I made just as much money as I did counting and enjoyed it more. I enjoyed counting, but I'm very lucky today because I hacked my own luck. I hope you do the same thing. I get to do what I love for a living, work with great people, and build wealth for the future, and no one wants to break my kneecaps for it.

CHAPTER **SUMMARY**

- Luck is not just about randomness. It's also more than where you are born or what DNA you have. Counting cards showed me that luck can be influenced by strategy.
- Define a win; don't be a perfectionist. You don't need to reach twenty-one, you just need to beat the dealer.
- Try to rush, and you'll make mistakes. Hacking timing often means waiting for the right time to strike.
- If you want to achieve something, look to others who have done it. It seems the more I learn, the luckier I get.
- Get where you want to go by giving others what they want, but make sure your skills and what you offer are what people want.
- Play with scale. Try things on a small scale with little risk; then, if it goes well, scale up.
- We think "win-win" means both sides win if a project is a success, but if you want to succeed, make plans that benefit you if they succeed or fail.
- The best way to plan ahead is to extend current trends. To do this we need to avoid ideological thinking and just read the data.

36 | Brain Fog

It was late 2020, in the COVID era. Lockdowns were in place, and vaccines were just being talked about. People finally realized this pandemic was going to last for a long time. I was working from home and had just pivoted my business to doing more online work. I was one of the fortunate ones who was doing well during this time.

We know the brain functions with the twin talents of memory and mirror. This means that most mental functions we perform can fall into the category of either recalling something or comparing something to others. From driving to dating, we are constantly recalling and comparing things to navigate this world, but what happens when you stifle these experiences and every day seems the same? The talent dulls and a fog rolls in.

One night, I was just about to drift off to sleep when I got a call from an old friend. "Dave? Is that you?" a frightened voice on the line said.

I checked the call display. It was from L.A. and from a man I hadn't talked to in years. Leon.

I met him back when I did seminars on memory in L.A. and San Diego. That was a great time. My workshops were *packed*, and I was able to help thousands of people. It even led to some amazing experiences like working with Forest Whitaker, who, in my opinion, is one of the best actors in Hollywood today.

Leon made an impression on me. He was passionate about applying brainhacks to his work. He memorized the names of people he worked with in his insurance company and kept learning on the job. He said it helped his career and even got him a promotion in the insurance company. Now he sounded like a spy running from foreign agents.

"Nice to hear from you," I said, "but it's kind of late over here with the time difference. I'm on eastern time, so 8:30 p.m. in California is 11:30 p.m. on the East Coast."

"Sorry to bother you. I thought you would have forgotten me, but of course, you're the memory guy," he said, wandering around in his speech. "That's what I want to talk about . . ." At this point, he broke into tears, which he seemed to have been holding in. "I think I'm losing my mind! I can't remember anything anymore!"

That phrase always sends a chill down my spine. I remember my grandmother developing Alzheimer's and needing round-the-clock care. Then, she got sick. As she lay there dying, her treatment was complicated by the disease. I remember her look of confusion and fear when the doctors and nurses were trying to help her. She didn't know what was happening at the end. They tried to save her body, but her mind was already gone. I pushed these thoughts away.

I told him that if he thinks he's losing his memory, it's a good sign, because Alzheimer's covers its tracks. There's a morbid joke about Alzheimer's that neuroscientists tell. Not to be mean, but as an explanation to others. They say that the patients actually have it easier because they forget they have a disease. It's funny because it's true. One of the symptoms of Alzheimer's is that you don't think you have a problem with your memory. As the brain covers its tracks, the forgetful forget they're sick.

This makes it extra tough for loved ones. As a result, most people diagnosed with dementia are dragged to the doctors by their worried families. At first, they're in denial because they don't think they have a problem, even though they may have sixteen containers of cream going bad in their fridge. After all, they need it for their morning coffee.

Leon breathed a sigh of relief but doubled down on his concern. "Well, I have this terrible brain fog. After three months into the COVID lockdowns, I noticed that I can't remember anything and can't focus. I'm depressed, and it's only getting worse. So, I went to the doctor, and they sent me home because they had bigger problems. Do you have any suggestions?" he pleaded.

Distant Shadow Memory Hack

Remember the Exploding Keys Brainhack? It helps to find lost items if you ask questions about how they look. The same concept, when combined with a journal, can recreate long-lost memories and even fight brain fog and memory loss. I first developed this for my (now late) great uncle Mike, who served in WWII. Over the decades since the war, he forgot the names of some he served with. But after doing this exercise, he was able to recall some and then find out what happened to them after the war.

Step One: Get a book with lined paper.

Step Two: Write down what you want to remember. Things from your childhood, the name of someone, where you buried that computer with Bitcoin codes in it.

Step Three: Go to sleep.

Step Four: First thing in the morning after you wake up, try to answer the question.

Step Five: Try again. At first, you won't recall anything. Then, you'll remember the information about what you are looking for, like where you met someone but not their name. Then, over time, you'll recall more. The information is in there somewhere. This can be a fun and rewarding exercise that brings back pleasant memories while training your brain.

This hit close to home. Not because he was a friend or customer but because I had the same symptoms and had been in denial until I heard it from him. I hadn't told anyone. Being the memory guy is like being the fastest gun in the West. You can't admit that you may be fallible. In reality, I may have trained my brain, but I'm still subject to problems from stress, overwork, and modern challenges. It took COVID to make me see cracks in my own ability, and I know if I was suffering, others had it much worse.

BRAIN FOG DEFINED

Brain fog is considered a syndrome, not a medical condition; however, it can be a symptom of another disease like MS, chronic fatigue syndrome (CFS), thyroid issues, and low testosterone. So, if you're worried about this, tell your doctor.

It comes on suddenly and can last any amount of time. Often, brain fog involves a combination of things—stress, loss of energy or sex drive, memory loss, cognitive decline, and/or lack of good judgment, to name a few.

Hack the Dumbing Down from Smart Phones

It has long been known that reliance on technology hurts our brains. Smartphones are slowly making us dumb. It's a phenomenon called the Google effect. Since the '70s, when we started to record memory ability, test results worldwide have gone down. For example, in North America, people have gone from being able to recall a list of seven things on average (that's why a phone number is seven digits long) to only four or five. The reason has been linked to technology. Since we no longer need to hold numbers and dates in our heads, we've gotten lazy. This has created a dramatic rise in incidences of brain fog. The hack for this is simple. Do all the brainhacks in this book. Take action. The brain loves to learn new things.

More severe cases can show symptoms like difficulty separating objects visually from a distance, irritability, insomnia, headaches, dizzy spells, inflammation, depression, intestinal or stomach problems, and weight gain.

Doctors blame work, stress, hormones, lack of sleep, modern lifestyles, lousy diet, and pollution. Throw in a dash of international pandemic and political divides, and you get severe brain fog that lasts a lot longer.

As a result, these days, many people feel like zombies in a constant state of fogginess, triggered by hormone changes like those that show up in women after giving birth and during menopause.

Before you think men get off easy, they have brain fog in record numbers in middle age. In addition, some studies show that, on average, middle-aged women outperform men on cognitive tests.

My personal theory is that men get brain fog less often but live with it longer because it doesn't come with a change in life like pregnancy or menopause, and men are less likely to visit a doctor, so they suffer without treatment.

Friendly note to the men reading: Go to the doctor. Statistically, there is probably something wrong with you right now that you're not addressing.

Combatting Brain Fog Hacks

The first step before we hack the brain is to *feed* the brain. It's easy to forget the brain is an organ in the body, so it needs nutrients and oxygen. Instead, think of the brain as the greedy organ, taking far more oxygen and fuel than other organs of the same size. It's like the Hummer of the biological highway.

Combatting Inflammation—Since inflammation is linked to brain fog, the best first step to lower inflammation is cutting out sugar and inflammatory oils like corn and vegetable oil. Basically, things that did not exist a thousand years ago are probably not ideal for your body today. A powerful machine needs to run on good fuel.

Exercise—This also increases blood flow and oxygen levels. Regular exercise has a knock-on effect that will benefit too many areas of your life to list here. It would take less time to describe the parts of the body that exercise doesn't help. I was about to say the hair and fingernails but turns out regular exercise improves both of these. Not to split hairs, of course.

Nutrition—Get all your nutrients with a balanced diet and even multivitamins. Some diets have been linked to brain fog—for example, when people fully cut out things like carbs or protein or restrict dietary variety, brain fog becomes more likely. Brain fog is also often triggered by hormone changes, and a good diet will help balance hormones.

Be Social—This is a common way to fight Alzheimer's and has shown promise in combatting brain fog and general cognitive challenges. Humans are essentially social creatures, so meeting new people, interacting, and learning about other people seems to be the most challenging cognitive task. Think about it from the perspective of a computer. We've taught computers to outthink us at chess and a million other things, but they still can't do something as simple as holding a conversation. Because it's not simple; it actually stimulates the brain more than you think. It also makes us feel good and has a number of other benefits.

Sleep Better—Bad sleep can hurt our brain's ability to function. Irregular sleep throws our hormones out of balance, and sleep apnea (lack of oxygen) caused by blockages while sleeping can be very serious. If you snore, do something about it. Talk to your doctor, or as I did, change your sleep position.

Leon also told me how his brain fog got worse when he felt inflammation and achy joints, something I had experienced firsthand.

Using a double-blind testing procedure, Dr. Leonie Balter, working with the University of Birmingham's Centre for Human Brain Health, recently discovered a link between inflammation and alertness triggers in the brain. So, like in Alzheimer's, fighting inflammation may be preventative.

I gave Leon a list of treatments to fight brain fog based on the latest research, plus a few fun activities that I came up with that could help. All the while, I was thinking to myself that I needed to follow my own advice.

RARITY AND TRANSFERENCE

I saved the best treatment for brain fog until the end because it shows why brainhacks are more than just tricks. But in order to understand how novel activities work, I need to start with two principles of neuroscience: rarity and transference.

Remember the Rarity Axiom for memory techniques? The brain responds most to unique imagery. Well, turns out it works for things beyond just visualization. Your brain thrives on new information.

Novel Brain Training—Novel activities are things that challenge the brain. A wave of brain training apps on the market over the last ten years promised to improve cognitive function; however, research showed that they often caused a decline. The reason is that the brain needs new tasks. Once you get good at something, you don't need to make new connections.

Try brushing your teeth with the wrong hand, standing on one foot during a commercial break, or using memory techniques to learn a new language or skill.

Transference—I tell people that sudoku and crosswords will make you better at sudoku and crosswords and not much else. The brain seems to be very compartmentalized. Just think of all the techniques we needed to go over to improve memory. Each technique dealt with a different situation, and mastering has minimal effect on others. Fighting brain fog, however, seems to be the one exception to the rule. As long as you try new challenges and learn new skills, they will all help lift the brain fog. We believe that brain fog is a total brain phenomenon and stimulating one part helps wake it all back up.

* * *

The COVID-19 pandemic has been tragic in many ways, but mental alertness is one casualty people don't talk about.

All the solutions above (diet, social interaction, and better sleep) were blocked by restrictions and isolation, causing the big storm front of brain fog to roll over the entire world, and some didn't recover. Isolation in particular can trigger this condition. I learned in my work that brain fog can linger long after the cause is gone. Women for example report terrible brain fog after pregnancy or menopause. It's persistent and stays long after the event is over. This is where brainhacking comes in.

FOG NEEDS A KICK

Brain fog seems to come in and take hold. It doesn't leave on its own. It needs to be kicked out. The only way I have seen it go away is from intense stimulation with unique activities. I sat down with a deck of cards and tried to memorize it, failing at first. It was so difficult. My brain was clouded. But I kept trying. My favorite undertaking is to learn new skills, so I dove more into my robotics project and did all the other things on the list of treatments, from sleep to diet adjustments.

After just a couple of weeks, I felt like a new man. The forgetfulness was gone, along with the irritability and stress. Every day seemed a little brighter. I checked in with Leon, and he was excited.

"I'm feeling so much better! I tried brushing my teeth with the wrong hand and exercising, and it worked. My brain is back!"

After my bout with brain fog, I was feeling better. But when the fog lifts, you'll notice things you didn't see before. What I noticed made my heart sink. My son had fallen deep into brain fog too and was really hurt by the isolation that sheltering in place for a year caused. I felt powerless and worried that isolation at this age could have permanent effects. COVID lockdowns have created a generation of cognitive regression that we will only truly understand years from now.

Working long hours, I'd been ignoring him. Brain fog also caused behavioral problems for him. He was bouncing off the walls (sometimes literally) and acting out. I gave him the nickname Xiao Huangdi, which means "little emperor" in Chinese (a nickname many Chinese kids get when acting out, since the old one-child policy created a generation of spoiled single children).

I'd like to say I sat down and did some memory tricks, which made him feel better, but it's not that simple. Instead, we worked hard to get him to connect on social media with others and spent a long vacation at my parents' cottage before he returned to school.

When school started back up, we tried to return to a new normal, but he was so far behind that homework sometimes gave him headaches: a physical example of his difficulty in handling information that was both too challenging and not stimulating enough. I decided to take more breaks and just play with him, and that made all the difference. After that, he started to feel better and do better in school.

One time when we were playing, he asked, "Daddy, will I catch up from COVID?"

I was shocked that he was so self-aware of his challenges. He had probably overheard my wife and me worriedly talking about how his reading skills had fallen behind.

At that moment, newfound confidence came over me. Thinking back to the challenges I'd faced and the uphill battle I had won against the system and my diagnosis, I realized he would have it much better than me. He was already catching up and had the makings to be anything he wanted to be. I smiled because the goal of any parent is for their children to have a better life than them.

"You'll catch up in no time. You've already gotten better in just a few months, and as you get older, I'll teach you all the brainhacks I know so you can ace your studies," I said.

He hugged me, and we kept playing.

CHAPTER **SUMMARY**

- The Distant Shadow Memory Hack can help you recall old, forgotten memories and can combat brain fog.
- Your smartphone is making you dumber. Take regular breaks from the tiny computer in your pocket and your brain will thank you.
- The best way to combat brain fog is to feed your brain what it needs to function at its best: take steps to decrease inflammation, exercise more, eat well, maintain healthy relationships, and get better sleep, and all the brainhacks in this book will be easier.

37 | Destination Setting

"Find out who you are and do it on purpose."

—Dolly Parton

I was running my business in Toronto when I got the news. My Guinness Record was broken again—by Dominic O'Brien, the guy who I won it from before. Dominic got the energy up ten years after I broke the record first to take it back.

My honest reaction was that he impressed me. I admired his skill and thought someone would have broken the record sooner anyway. However, the timing was bad for me.

I had started to work in technology and design as a passion, but that did not pay the bills yet, and my memory business had slowed down. Many of the places I was traveling to had seen me before, so the market was becoming saturated. People who had taken my seminar were happy but didn't need it again. I tried to travel more and still did well in interviews, but I was treading water. Then, after years of doing business across the border, I was stopped and turned around before a major media tour. The lawyers said it shouldn't have happened, but the damage was done. I lost months of business and thousands of dollars. There is no straight line to business success. Although my jump into technology was a distraction, there was no way to go back in time, so I had to go forward.

I needed to change this around. Thankfully, as you may guess, there is a brainhack for this. In my first memory course, I added a concept called "destination setting." Think of it as a more powerful form of goal setting and the culmination of all the principles I have taught so far. It combines the strategies of luck hacks and future hacks with the success technique of visualization and the organization of the Journey Brainhack. Now was the time to use it.

Many people in the self-help world talk about manifesting something they want. We have all heard of the law of attraction and the belief that focus and drive can direct your life. But it's also natural to be skeptical because there is little evidence for it. Most social scientists will tell you manifestation is simply the survivorship bias. If many people try something and only a few succeed, then those who succeed think they're special.

Also, can you really say someone achieved their goal when any study of success shows it takes a lot of failures to get to one success? So, maybe I had a good run, and now it was time to try something else? Get further into technology? Or marketing?

The only problem with the skepticism around setting goals or aiming for success is that it does not match the facts. This has been studied time and again and in every area of human achievement. From kids learning musical instruments to professional athletes, those who set and, yes, try to manifest goals, outperform those who don't. Not once or twice but consistently. It will please the skeptics to know that this doesn't mean that those who set goals manifest everything they aim for—far from it. Even untrained negative-thinking people who are told to set goals for a psychology study outperform those who don't.

The power of goal setting is the legacy of the amazing mind we all have. Our brain is a problem solver, a survival tool, and all it needs is direction to bring out its best. It's often said that aiming for a goal doesn't mean you will hit it, but you will miss every shot you never try.

WHAT IS WRONG WITH GOAL SETTING?

That said, there are a few things I didn't like about modern goal-setting advice. First, the idea of a goal is to stand in one place and aim for a target. Life is about more than just hitting a target. It also implies that someone in the way (a goalie) wants to stop you. Since images have always helped me, I wanted to visualize my goals. Still, this process of aiming at something through the obstacles didn't motivate me or bring about creative ideas to solve problems. It felt empty, like I would aim at a number, hit that target, then start all over the next day. There was no feeling of progress. This is part of the positive thinking cycle that many see as almost toxic in that it focuses people's attention on hitting a number and not building a better life. Plus, all the data showed that it wasn't just the goals that helped people achieve something. A *plan* is pivotal. So, saying someone can achieve something simply by setting a goal is an oversimplification.

I decided that most people think of goal setting as a sport—aiming for a goal. But I wanted something more . . . like the process used to win a battle or land an airplane. I wanted a process to create a powerful, effective plan to get me from point A to point B. So, I didn't want a goal; I wanted a destination.

WORKING BACKWARD

Imagine you're on a plane sitting on the tarmac when the pilot comes over the speaker and says, "Good afternoon, ladies and gentlemen. Our goal today is to get to Hawaii! I'm really motivated and will work very hard, so I think we can get there this time."

Everyone would get off that plane. So, why do we treat our lives this way? I discovered the solution is to work backward. Our brains are much better at creative thinking if we are looking back rather than forward, even if it's a hypothetical situation.

The analogy of a plane actually works perfectly. Here's what I mean: The trip of a major airliner is planned in reverse. Experts start the plan by picking and understanding the destination, then make sure the airport will be ready for us to land when we want to arrive. Then, they work backward, getting clearance for weather and air routes along the way, calculating the amount of fuel needed and departure times. Finally, they check in passengers and inspect the plane before leaving. They don't just get in the air, aim at the destination, and work hard.

I used to be guilty of the ready-fire-aim mentality. When I started, I would often just jump into a new venture, then figure it out as I went. But my more successful ventures came about when I started to employ backward planning. Interestingly, I'm told many successful launches use this same backward-planning principle. It was even taught at Harvard for making effective business plans.

Destination Setting Brainhack

Step One: Pick the destination.

Step Two: Visualize it; make it real.

Step Three: Ask questions to paint the picture.

Step Four: Make it now.

Step Five: At each stage, mentally look back and ask yourself, *How did I get here?* Let your mind answer.

Step Six: Step back to the big milestone just before the current image. Repeat the process, and ask questions to paint a picture. Think of it as the present moment, and ask yourself how you arrived at this point.

Step Seven: Write down the steps you took on the way back— every milestone and every solution you used to get over it.

Join me in the next exercise where we turn your goals into destinations and your dreams into plans.

DESTINATION SETTING EXERCISE

Step One: Pick the destination. This may sound easy because everyone wants the same things—money, power, happiness, love. Pick the basic outcome that you truly want. In reality, this is the most difficult thing to do. You need to be specific. That's where the next steps come in.

Step Two: Visualize it; make it real. More than a picture. Use all your senses and imagine you are walking through the house of your dreams or spending time with the family you hope to have, or attending the graduation of your child. As you know, the power of visualization works to get your brain focused. So, take a moment and imagine as many aspects as possible of this perfect life you want.

Step Three: Ask questions to paint the picture. This gets the brain involved in making the destination real. For example, ask your brain what your house looks like. Do you have pets? Who are you with? Who loves you? Ask if you have kids or where you want to live. Right down to what the floor looks like, tile or carpet—ask all the questions you can. If you get your brain to help make the destination, it feels real. Also, be open to change. When I stared asking questions, my mind told me to move to the States from Canada. I didn't think of that until I asked myself the open-ended questions. The answers told me I had to work with a major US corporation and move to the USA.

Step Four: Make it now. Imagine this is real in the present moment. This will be a real meta moment because you know it's a future event you are thinking of, but for some reason the brain does not really take it seriously if it's hypothetical. It has to be happening now to be real. This is the toughest thing to do because you imagine something that you see in the future by default. But if you can imagine that it already exists in the present moment, the results will be much greater. So, take a moment and imagine everything happening on today's date. I imagine a calendar on the wall or a live broadcast on the TV.

I wasted years visualizing plans that were always two years in the future, and that is where they stayed. I was always two years away from the goal. When I switched to imagining things I already wanted to be in my life, everything changed.

Step Five: Look back. Now that you have a clear idea of your destination, ask yourself, *How did I get here? What step would have brought me here?* Again, your brain will answer the question, and it may surprise you. The answer will help create a guide map to reach this destination. Take a lot of notes as you meditate on this. What you are looking for is to paint a picture of the step just before the final step. I call this your milestones. Success does not happen overnight. There are steps to a plan. Flesh out each step.

Step Six: Repeat the process until you get back to the present. Write down the steps you took on the way back—every milestone and every solution you used to get over it.

* * *

When anyone does a goal-setting workshop or a life plan like this, they walk away with a bunch of notes. Really dig deep into this process. When I did it back then, the notes I made amazed me. It was a step-by-step plan to get the life I wanted. Every milestone fit and made sense from beginning to end, although I had no idea how I would accomplish them. Here are some highlights:

- The first step on the way to my destination was to get back into the Guinness Record books.
- After I get the record, I would do more business in America with a work visa or green card.
- I also saw my girlfriend taking a larger role in my business and personal life.
- I wrote down that I would need to work with a major corporation and get national media attention.
- If I was going to have this dream life, I needed to master marketing, and I imagined hiring a team to do my marketing and grow that part of the business.
- I wanted to speak in front of crowds but had no idea how, so one milestone was to build a professional speaking career.

- I also wanted to get back into technology but in the field of robotics. I honestly didn't know the applications, but I felt like that was a piece of the plan.

After looking at the plan, I made it into a meditation of sorts. it reminded me of things I told Mr. Ross years ago. I wanted to get into marketing, run a business, and speak to crowds.

I hadn't thought about that for years, but visualizing the destination brought out my deepest thoughts. I knew I was on the right track, but I still wasn't prepared for the massive change ahead.

Starting off, I needed to go for that record. So, I did a destination-setting plan for just that goal. I imagined I had accomplished it and asked how I reached each milestone and solved each problem. It was amazing how easy it was to think of great ideas simply by putting myself in the perspective of hindsight.

THE RECALL

It was the early 2000s and I had learned from my past experience. The attempt actually went smoothly this time. One of the ideas that came to me in my meditation was to use my old high school as the venue for breaking the record. The Guinness Books required people of standing in the community as witnesses (teachers fit that), and this seemed like the best place to do it. It was bittersweet, though, because my friends weren't there. I felt Mr. Muller's absence in every hallway, and somehow everything was tiny. It's amazing what you notice when you get older. The halls had the same energy, though. It was the same high school where I'd had so many struggles with Mr. Ross. He was absent too, but I did recognize many of the teachers and others even recognized me.

My record of fifty-two decks had been broken with two more decks. So even though my record was broken, I felt like the new goal was attainable. I was planning to do ten decks more so it would stand again for a long time. But for some reason, when it came time to do the record, a few of the blue-backed decks turned out to be red when opened. I could not use them, and the number of decks was reduced to fifty-nine decks of cards (3,068 cards in total). The Guinness rules were very strict, but I had been through this rodeo before, so we were prepared.

The reason to use a good venue like the school or museum is that Guinness rules specifically require two upstanding members of the community to be present and sign forms proving they witnessed the event. So, apparently, we can't trust one upstanding community member, but two works. This means for a record like this, you need either two extremely dedicated people or many that rotate. The teachers really came through, and of course, they rotated shifts to shuffle all the cards and witness me memorize every card. I could only see each card once.

After the memorization phase was done, the plan was to move everything under lock and key to the discovery channel studios at CTV in Toronto for the recall. I learned from the last time how important it was to balance getting the most publicity I could out of this event while still keeping the media at arm's length, so I didn't make a mistake.

A few witnesses and friends sat in the green room with me for hours while I recited card after card. It was perfect—until deck seventeen. I said the seven of clubs when the card was actually the jack of clubs. (At the time, it was a weird dyslexia-inspired twist of the image in my head; if you flip a seven upside down, it looks similar to a J.) I didn't stress. In fact, I had planned for this. I had spent days doing event rehearsal and imagining what I would do when I made my first mistake. I walked a bit to clear my head and then returned and recited every other card perfectly to the end.

I broke the record, and it now stands at fifty-nine decks of playing cards memorized after seeing them only once with only one mistake. So, I guess all that effort training to eliminate errors worked.

It was amazing, and I'm forever grateful to everyone at Eastwood Collegiate School. Today, there is an article hanging on a wall in the school about the accomplishment. I have no idea who put it up, but it feels like my journey came full circle.

This was just the first step, though. The next major steps on my destination-setting plan were to get a work visa or green card for America. After that, I wanted to work with a major corporation and develop a marketing team around me. That way, I could help my business grow. Ultimately getting involved in technology again would also be wonderful.

Reader revolution.

After breaking the record for a second time, I made the news everywhere. It was amazing. By this time, I was an expert at getting PR and media attention for myself, and I leveraged it into many media appearances. Finally, someone must have been paying attention because a representative for Sony Corporation called to offer me the oddest thing I could have imagined.

They wanted me to sit in a Manhattan store front window, just a few blocks from Times Square, and speed-read for a PR stunt.

After finding out how much I would be paid for the event, I agreed quickly, and they covered my work visa. It was a nail-biting time waiting for the approval. It all came down to one deadline, when the team was about to pull the plug on the event entirely if the visa didn't show up within two days. I dove hard into the visualization techniques, hoping they would help manifest the result I needed.

I imagined the event happening, and all the other milestones to my destination being real. I can't say that the technique brought my dream into a reality because the visa took over four days longer. Well past the deadline. But being so focused did change how I came across over the phone. I was able to show such confidence that it bought the extra time needed. That meant that I accomplished two more of my milestones in one fell swoop.

FARROWBOT

There I was, sitting in the window display. People were walking to and from work while I sat on my Murphy bed. I thought, *Life can't get odder than this.*

I felt exposed. Every move I made caused people walking by to jump, not realizing a living human was in this window display. I was amazed by how people reacted to any movement. In that moment, I got the idea for a robot that would move in retail windows attracting customers. Later, I would turn this idea into a design and a new robotics startup, hitting another of my milestones.

There in the window, I felt unstoppable, until one day a guy in a trench coat and fedora hat came to the window with a sign. It said, "Are you Dave Farrow?" *This is it,* I thought. *This is the day I die.* I waited for him to pull out a gun. Was I paranoid? Or was it that no one wore fedoras and trench coats anymore? I'm basically advertising that I'm a sitting duck with media attention around me. Instinctually, though, I nodded, and he turned the sign around. It read, "Andrew Vachss sends his regards."

The author Andrew Vachss is a favorite of mine. He discovered what I was doing and asked his fan base to send me some love. The only issue is he is a crime writer so it nearly scared the crap out of me. Considering his novels are some of the best crime dramas I have ever read, it seemed fitting that my reaction would be one of mortal fear. I had to laugh. Good job.

The device I was promoting was Sony's attempt to enter the e-reader market. They had just developed the reader to compete with the Kindle. It was a shame the product didn't take off because Sony's device was better in so many ways. It allowed you to drag and drop PDFs and Word documents into it and allowed you to use multiple libraries and make notes while reading. But, of course, that was one of the problems. When you buy a Kindle, you get the Kindle library. At the time, Oprah was promoting the Kindle, and I was promoting the Sony reader, so it didn't take much effort to determine who would win that battle.

That said, it was a successful campaign. Both in my compensation and in the media coverage it got. I was featured on *Regis and Kelly, Dr. Oz,* and page six of the *New York Times,* to name a few. So, it was a powerful experience. It was also a historic time because it was 2008, and Obama had just been elected president. So, I got to engage in several interviews about the moment as a commentator, which was priceless.

PETITE

After the event was over, I had an odd meeting with the immigration lawyers. They told me that turning this temporary visa into a green card wouldn't be much work. Still, I would have to move to America for several years and not go back home to visit for a while.

I could write a book about the problems with America's immigration system. They had lots of weird rules. They asked me about Andrea, at the time my girlfriend, whom I called Petite as a pet name. If we got married, she could come with me, but it would basically be impossible to make it work otherwise. That was a lot to take in. I did think we were going to be together long-term. I wanted to spend my life with her. But we have an unorthodox relationship and never liked labels. So, my lawyers said it would either be a very short or very long conversation. She would either be very happy or very awkward.

I would either have to break up or get married, and if she chose to follow, she would need to stop everything and come with me in the next couple of weeks. At the time, Andrea was a certified high school teacher. She taught supply (in America, this is what is called substitute teaching) on a small school board but planned to go full time.

She had a life, family, and friends all in Canada, and nothing but me if she came to the United States. At the same time, she was growing disillusioned with teaching. She had been using memory techniques in classes and knew how effective they were. She got excited when she would teach a list technique and get a class to memorize twenty-one random items. The entire class would be able to remember them perfectly even when she returned months later. The students would talk about the learning tools, but the teachers didn't seem to care. She was passionate about education and wanted more.

I decided to broach the subject the next time I saw her.

"Hey, Petite. Can I talk to you for a sec?" I said softly.

Her Spidey-sense went off immediately. "What's wrong?" she said. "What happened? You don't talk to me like that unless something's wrong."

"Well, I guess I just need to explain the whole thing. I have a chance to turn my temporary work visa into a green card and go to America. It has a bigger market and a ton of opportunities for us—especially this memory business. But if we do this, we will need to get married and leave everything behind, starting over in the middle of a recession. So, I can't give any guarantees. In fact, it's very—"

"When do we go?" she interrupted.

"Really? You want to go and do this?" I replied, trying to hold back tears.

"Yes, but this isn't what I thought of when I imagined getting married so . . . a few rules. One: no emotions right now," she said, standing up, pointing at me. The emotion was building behind her façade, breaking her first rule already. "You didn't just propose to me; you still need to do that. You just explained a shared business opportunity."

"Okay, business partner," I said, emotional myself but playing along.

"And we get quickly hitched at City Hall and don't tell anyone until we can plan a big wedding because I don't want anyone to not show up to my wedding because of this."

"I agree to those terms," I answered, still playing it cool but trying to hold back tears.

Then, she jumped into my arms. Her dream in life was to make a bigger impact working with me than she ever could in one classroom in one school in one region, and she lived up to that. She took on the name Mrs. Memory and taught seminars herself while also doing sales and more. We got married at the courthouse and wouldn't tell anyone for two years because we wanted to have a proper ceremony after getting a chance to plan ahead. Then, we moved. Right into the biggest economic recession in US history—the 2008 housing crash.

So, what I was offering wasn't considered essential at the time—and it certainly wasn't in demand. I still worked hard, but those first few years were tough. My wife was there helping with sales while I would drive into New York and market myself, but it wasn't working. The core business was stale. More than that, more people were entering the memory world, and it was getting saturated. But the Sony event did yield some great results. I licensed my memory course to an infomercial company and got royalties on my product plus sales through media appearances. Then, I started speaking more and more. My biggest market was colleges. The boy who was told he wouldn't get past the gate except as a gardener was now being advertised as a guest speaker to help the students study.

Around that time, other authors came up to me in droves asking how I got so many media appearances. So, I started teaching PR, then doing one-on-one consulting, and finally hired a small team to take on clients. Suddenly, I was running a PR firm and reached another destination visualization milestone—to build a marketing team around me. Little did I know that this team would grow and become what many have called the most innovative PR company for authors in America today. Today, Farrow Communications is a full-service PR and marketing firm.

No matter what you want to accomplish, no career is out of a brain-hacker's reach. Years after living in a window for Sony, my PR firm was running smoothly, so I started thinking about getting back into technology. The experience in the window had made me think about technology from a different perspective. I remembered that every time I moved, people reacted. As it turns out, humans are wired to pay attention to humanoid shapes.

I have a dream that someday humans will live alongside humanoid robots like in Isaac Asimov's writing. Only, despite what Hollywood imagines, it would be symbiotic—like how pets live with and benefit us. I think this is inevitable. Turning to the destination-setting exercise, I asked myself what would have to happen before that step.

My answer was a non-walking humanoid robot. Useful long-lasting bipedal robotic walking still hasn't been created. (Most YouTube videos you see don't show the part where the robot runs out of energy in twenty-two minutes.) Then, I asked myself what we could do with a non-walking humanoid robot. It was obvious. Moving mannequins would work, so why weren't there animatronic (moving) mannequins? There were some fun art pieces but nothing affordable or common. If it could be built, it would change every retail store in the world. It would raise sales and bring in foot traffic. It would bring in customers and make shopping more fun.

Whoever builds the company to tackle this project better have a background in marketing and sales because they would essentially be salespeople. It would need PR to take advantage of media to market it, and it would require an out-of-the-box designer who could learn new technology fast. A line by Liam Neeson from *Taken* popped in my head: "I have . . . a very particular set of skills, skills I have acquired over a very long career."

FarrowBOT launches next year. Because life is meant to be lived on purpose.

All of these events happened one after the other, just the way I had seen when I asked my brain for guidance.

I have to admit I was hooked on destination setting. I have no need for anyone else to believe this. Still, I think the process played out so uncannily that it's some kind of evidence we are connected in some way.

I've seen enough data to think that we are all connected. That our thoughts influence others and the world around us. I don't believe we can just manifest anything, but we can influence things beyond what we think is possible. Even if this is not true, the idea is a useful belief. Carl Jung talked about all of humanity sharing a collective consciousness, and I think it's possible. I don't think everything happens for a reason because so many bad things happen to good people. But on some level, we *are* connected. We all are sharing information, and it results in two people inventing the same thing on different sides of the planet from time to time. Other times, it gives people the sense of being stared at, so they turn around just in time to catch the wandering eyes of another looking away. And sometimes it means making the goals you've set and made real through visualization come true. When this happens, things seem to fall into place as if they were guided there.

We humans, all of us on this planet, are interconnected—indeed, part of the same whole.

CHAPTER **SUMMARY**

- Instead of planning a goal, plan a destination and work backward from there.
- No matter what you want to do or accomplish, no career is out of a brainhacker's reach.

EPILOGUE: THE RECIPE

Thank you for reading *Brainhacker*. I hope you liked reading it as much as I liked writing it. I want to leave you with a very big idea that will be made into a future book. If you believe in the brainhacker's philosophy of personal improvement and growth, then this is an opportunity to use what you know to help others.

In this book, I have been critical of big organizations, wanting to see reform. It's easy to criticize though. I want to create a system to help organizations make better decisions. A kind of group brainhack.

Today, the way groups make decisions is flawed. If there is one leader, it's a dictatorship and can never rise above the intelligence or knowledge of that one person, missing out on the talent of everyone else.

Democracy outperforms that by giving a voice to people. That freedom means everyone gains from each other's talents. But, after being unfairly sentenced to death, Socrates best summed up the dangers of democracy as being a form of mob rule. Remember, a mob of people with pitchforks is a democracy too. So, we just traded the tyranny of the king for the tyranny of the mob or of the bureaucracy. There is one flaw in the current system:

We enforce laws based on evidence but create them based on opinion.

Whether it's the employee handbook, local bylaws, or even being accused of a crime in most developed nations, there is a trial or a process that weighs evidence before arriving at a decision.

But the rules and laws themselves are not held to the same standard. We don't hold laws to the same standard that we enforce them with. There is no burden of proof to create a law. Corruption, money, mob mentality, ideology, propaganda, and groupthink can influence the process. Running a PR firm, I see firsthand how public opinion on a subject can be changed with the right spin.

We need to create laws based on evidence and proof rather than opinion.

We need a better system so that all the effort now put into propaganda and fake conspiracies would be used for evidence gathering and working out the math.

I started to ask myself how to create a "practical system™" like this and I came up with a game.

I call it "The Recipe™" because it allows people who disagree to input their facts and evidence (the ingredients), and the game bakes those details and helps them arrive at a beautiful conclusion. It helps large and small groups make better decisions and fair laws by using simple math and data, not opinion, to provide real answers to tough questions.

I am still working on the details, and that's where you come in.

I have already created some of the principles and posted them—things like the "Math of Things," where issues can be given a numeric value, and the "Pillars of Truth," about how options can be weighed in a pro and con method showing which idea wins.

I plan to develop this into a method any organization can use to run better, and I want your help.

Join me at *brainhackers.com*, and take part in the discussions. Lend your voice and let's start to make history. You can also dive deeper into more fun brainhacks from other experts and become a contributor yourself. Do this by joining the hundreds of experts who have already contributed content.

If you enjoyed this book, the best way to thank me is to use these hacks.

Live life on purpose and encourage society to think critically about the decisions we make.

Together, we can be smarter, healthier, and happier, thinking more clearly and grasping goals by taking charge of the gray matter between our ears.

Don't let this be the end of your journey but the beginning of it.

ABOUT THE AUTHOR

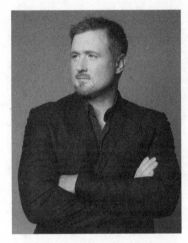

Dave Farrow is the two-time Guinness World Record holder for greatest memory. To earn this title, Farrow recalled the exact order of 59 decks of shuffled playing cards using "The Farrow Memory Method." This method was originally invented to combat Farrow's dyslexia and ADHD and it is now a unique memory system backed by a double-blind neuroscience study from McGill University.

Farrow has been a featured guest expert on more than 2,000 interviews, including multiple appearances on *The Dr. Oz Show, TODAY, Live with Regis and Kelly, The Steve Harvey Show,* Discovery Channel, and many others. Today, Farrow uses his keen understanding of the brain in the public relations and media sector. He is the CEO of Farrow Communications, a full-service PR firm known for memorable marketing.

PREVIEW FOR MY NEXT BOOK

HOW TO FORGET

My next book, *How to Forget*, started as a joke when people used to come up to me in seminars asking how to forget things like their ex-spouse or a terrible movie. But soon, this idea turned into something more. I talked to victims of trauma who were working hard to forget the past and forge a brighter future. I spoke with couples' counselors who see the suffering caused in relationships by people who refuse to let go of grudges or baggage. If our brains were houses, we would all be hoarders of old negative thoughts that don't serve us anymore. What are you holding on to that you would like to forget?

The Forgetting Hack

One time, I was involved in an accident with a pedestrian. To be more specific, my stopped car was involved in the accident. A man was crossing the road when another vehicle in the opposing lane of traffic hit him and threw him into the side of my car. I remember seeing his face just before he crashed into my driver's side door. The paramedics took him away. Despite having received every assurance that he was uninjured, I couldn't get his face out of my head. I replayed the crash over and over in my dreams, too, haunted by it. Until I decided to skip the record.

Skip the Record

Step One: Imagine the traumatic event from beginning to end or at least as much of it as you can.

Step Two: Imagine it again but change something that makes it less scary, like adding music or putting a silly costume on people.

Step Three: Repeat this again and again, visualizing the event more and more, making it funnier or stranger. This process is a way to emotionally take back that event by gaining control. But it also twists the very memory of the event itself to the point where most can't even recall the original image.

Step Four: Take it further. What others in the past didn't realize is that you can do this for all kinds of things you want to let go of (e.g., relationship baggage and minor grudges). It's a tool that allows you to let go and move on. The power is in your hands to make this change.

THE REASON WE FORGET

In the past, I thought the reason we forget was that we are imperfect. I thought that forgetting was a mistake of the brain. But the truth is that the brain has the capability for near-perfect recall. We know this because of the tremendous results from memory training but also from outliers. Many people have been identified by science to have near-perfect recall of their lives through a condition called hypermnesia.

Now, we all want a better memory, so these people should be on cloud nine, but interestingly a study of these rare people who can recall every detail of their lives revealed a life of depression and loneliness. They found it almost impossible to have friends or romantic partners because they would never be surprised; they always knew things their partner didn't. In short, they didn't need others to survive.

When I compare this to a study of couples over seventy, a pattern becomes clear: When quizzed separately, these people had well below average recall of events from their past, and their memory became weaker over time. However, when quizzed as a couple, they scored much higher than younger single people in the same test. Their answers to questions were like a tennis game of back-and-forth communication where each half would recall a piece of the memory but neither one had the whole picture.

I think we forget so that we need to rely on others to get by. Being bonded together as a group is more important for our survival than any individual aptitude for memory.

So our memory is just good enough to avoid danger but bad enough to bring us together to help each other.

Don't let this be the end of your brainhacker journey but the beginning.

When I started my journey as a brainhacker, I wanted to unleash powers and fix my brain. Over time I have learned to do this but also appreciate the imperfect tool that is the human mind. Even things we think are flaws turn out to have purpose. What do you need to forget to grow as a person and what flaw could you turn into an advantage?